T0077915

WISDOM OF YOGA
PATH TO ASCENSION

GURU
BHANESHWARANAND

BALBOA.PRESS
A DIVISION OF HAY HOUSE

Balboa Press books may be ordered through booksellers or by contacting:

Balboa Press
A Division of Hay House
1663 Liberty Drive
Bloomington, IN 47403
www.balboapress.com
844-682-1282

Edited by Fabiana Bertolani

Print information available on the last page.

ISBN: 978-1-9822-6571-7 (sc)
ISBN: 978-1-9822-6570-0 (e)

Balboa Press rev. date: 05/04/2021

CONTENTS

Introduction vii

Chapter 1   Yama (Restrains) - Actions we should avoid 1

Chapter 2   Niyama (Observances) - Actions we should
            engage in 18

Chapter 3   Asanas (Postures) 34

Chapter 4   Pranayama (Breathing Techniques) 83

Chapter 5   Pratyahara (Withdrawal of the Senses) 123

Chapter 6   Dharana (Conceptualization or Concentration). . . . 128

Chapter 7   Dhyana (Meditation). 133

Chapter 8   Samadhi (Meditative state) 137

A day in the Life of Yogi 141

Conclusion 143

INTRODUCTION

All bliss is attainable in this lifetime, we can have it all. Everything we want is available and accessible to any of us. Tapping into that inner sea of abundance and wellbeing is the key.

How can we achieve all our heart's desires and fulfillment? It is NOT done through philosophy, religion or a belief system. It is achievable through the science and technology of yoga and spirituality. Yes you heard right, yoga is an ancient science, a technology that provides us the keys to powerful and valuable tools. We can arrive at a place where we feel we have it all, simply by taking advantage of the knowledge and reaching an understanding of how to walk the path.

This book has a dual purpose. On the one hand it helps all those desiring and willing to advance on their spiritual journey and on the other hand it is a guide for every human being to lead a healthier and blissful life.

We are "life force" living a human experience. Therefore, this book covers both, the physical as well as the spiritual aspects of our lives. I have outlined the complete and detailed path to follow for the ascension process in which we "de-identify" with the body and merge with the broader part of who we really are. This is done through the unlearning of all the limiting beliefs we have picked up along the trail of our life, debilitating patterns of behavior and habitual states of emotion that don't serve us. I will guide you through a step by step process where we master our thoughts, emotions and compulsions, so our innate intelligence works for us and not against us.

Ultimately the knowledge compiled here will strengthen the readers' capacity to reach and attain unification with the "divine essence" or what we call Source. As every human being's goal is to unify all aspects of the self with the Higher Self.

While some chapters will be geared more towards the physicality of our being others will explore the various states of consciousness. As we progress through the chapters it will be evident that it is mostly external work up to the chapter where we discuss pranayama, then once we have mastered the body we move along as we are equipped for the spiritual advancement leading us to the revered place of liberation or ascension, liberation being the final destination. As you break the cycle of life and death, you are liberated, not needing any further human experiences to complete any additional karma created; good nor bad.

In my years as a teacher and spiritual guide I have been asked the same question day in and day out. What can I do to feel better? I try to explain to my students that there is a presence in everyone's life consuming all their life energy. It is an energy we could consider a "negative" force which has overtaken humanity's capacity to be happy. This evil culprit, for those who love Star Wars can be compared to the "dark side".

Let's look at a simple example, Mr Y who wants to become an engineer, doctor, lawyer or businessman and goes through the struggles of application and finally getting accepted to the university of his choice. Are his struggles over? No! He completes his degree and, after acquiring his diploma and graduating gets the job of his dreams.... Are his challenges over? No! Now his objective is to earn a hundred thousand dollars. He works and strives and finally makes it. Is his torture over? No! This is an everlasting cycle with no end.

This evil force called "struggle" needs to be addressed and overcome. This book is here to assist in the dismantling of this unseen force which should have no power or grasp over our lives. The content is meant to provide tools that enable us to perceive reality in a different light so that we no longer merely react to life in a compulsive manner nor fall victim to our circumstances. My true hope is that it will alleviate the feeling of suffocation most people feel, therefore replacing that feeling of struggle with a sense of thriving in all areas of life. We are meant to have beautiful relationships, optimal health, abundant finances and a blissful existence.

The universe is on our side one hundred percent of the time. It is always assisting us in achieving our goals, calling us to follow our true nature which is to be at ease. In the process of creation, that is how life was intended to be. When we veer from our nature, we lose our inert sense of harmony and dis-ease takes hold.

This evil force of struggle is so present and so detrimental, we might as well consume small doses of poison on a daily basis and then wonder why we feel miserable. When people achieve their goals it is commonly short-lived, for an instant they are "struggle free" and then the feeling is overthrown with the need to "struggle" again. Humanity lives under the false premise that life must be difficult, that we must prove our worth. We don't realize it and fuel this subconscious need to be in a constant state of struggle as we even miss struggling when we notice it's absence. There is an unconscious belief that we must endure in order to achieve greatness, money, happiness like the saying says: "No pain, No Gain". We will "not knowingly" create scenarios that will most likely cause these emotions to arise on repeat. Unbeknownst to us we vibrate at a certain frequency in our ignorance and because we are under this illusory state of being we don't realize we have been programmed to suffer, to focus on the aspects of our life that are "not working" as we have a very negatively skewed vision of success. This "need to succeed" only keeps humans looping in a bad cycle that binds the person to an undesired energy of misery. What if instead we woke up in the morning and focused our attention on all the aspects that are working out well for us, we have a functioning body, warm water to bathe, food to nurture our cells and the potential to achieve every desire we could possibly have.

That is where the beauty of wisdom lies, better said the technology here presented becomes so relevant. Once we gain understanding and awareness of the laws of the universe, the toolset given here bridges *you to a state of calmness, satisfaction and gratitude which are the key components to attracting the life of our dreams.*

The emotion of satisfaction that shall prevail as our state of being will override any "need for success", hence eliminating the subconscious need to struggle. We will have the perception of already having attained it all, and therefore it shall be so. It can be no other way, when we are in the flow of life everything we desire has to make its way to us.

Through our yoga practice we achieve this feeling of satisfaction, we feel on top of the world like having achieved everything we need, liberated from any further compulsive urges; this feeling of utter stillness and peace generated from within gives meaning to an already fulfilled life.

Completeness is defined when we are one with all. We become enveloped in the sense of having reached heaven on earth. The truth is that we have consciously generated the feeling and created this reality from within, that shields us from any external discomfort. This state of being frees us from any outsourced need. We are finally in the driver's seat, having updated our software. We realize that we are the sole providers of our own bliss in this earthly experience.

What Is YOGA?

Yoga is connecting us to Source at which point we feel a sense of calmness and completeness.

Yoga (योग) is a physical, mental and spiritual process that transforms us from self to higher self and combines Atma (Soul) with Param Atma (Source). It has been known through eternity as a tool to reach perfection and completion. Its main goal is the attainment of a flawless state of spiritual alignment with Source. It is a process which, when performed correctly and by following the system of all eight limbs of Yoga (which is what we will be covering in this book), allows the person to connect to Source or their higher self.

Regular practice of Yoga helps to cultivate a strict discipline in eating habits, cleanliness, sexuality and character, thus enabling an individual to become a more evolved human being.

The therapeutic benefit of yoga is widely known and practiced worldwide. It is a fact that today yoga is considered a global phenomenon and an essential part of modern civilisation. However, yoga, like any other discipline when practiced in the wrong manner, and without professional guidance, can sometimes have adverse effects and therefore it is recommended to always be practiced under proper guidance.

It is of equal importance when practicing yoga to consider the appropriate amount of time, the place, the attire and mainly our diet. Yoga has to be practiced in a quiet, secluded place, in which fresh air is easily available - like a veranda, terrace, garden, etc. Ideally, yoga should be practiced in the early hours of either morning or evening on a relatively empty stomach.

However, it can be practiced either four hours after a heavy meal, or 20 minutes after a glass of juice or a cup of skimmed milk. On completion, one can have a meal after half-an-hour. Avoid tea, coffee, smoking, alcohol and spices.

The length of the practice should be adjusted to one's capacity. Most importantly, yoga should be practiced at the same time every day; in two sessions if one feels able. One may experience an initial stiffness of the limbs and muscles. This will ease with regular practice. During yoga, the attire has to be clean, light and loosely fitting to allow free movement; preferably light cotton garments. In cold climates, a shirt or thin sweater can also be used. To avoid discomfort, jewelry or accessories need to be taken off. One must always practice barefoot to ensure contact with the ground. Further, since the body has to be stretched in various directions, yogic practice has to be done on a clean mat, rug, carpet or a blanket. The seat should be firm and comfortable. Yoga should not be practised on any sofa surface.

During Yogasana (this will be explained in the Asana chapter), one should breathe through the nostrils and not through the mouth, except when it is mentioned to breathe through the mouth like in the case of Sheetali and Sheetkari Pranayama. While bathing is not directly related to yogasana, a shower before and after yogasana can refresh the body and mind.

Yoga should be commenced, in a calm, tension-free meditative posture. Be mindful to be in complete silence during the practice. One must not perform asanas during acute illnesses like fever, a severe asthmatic attack or extreme fatigue. Very weak patients in a state of extreme exhaustion should avoid holding the breath (Kumbhaka) during pranayama.

While in most physical exercises we lose energy to the universe, Yogic exercises are meant to achieve the exact opposite by attracting energy from the universe. That's why Yoga cools our bodies rather than making us sweat. We should never work up a sweat during yoga. Should it still happen, we should avoid wiping ourselves with a towel, instead it is advisable to rub the body with the palms of our hands. The sequence of yogic practices, i.e., Kriyas (work), Asanas (posture), Pranayama (breathing exercises), Chittashuddhi (purification of mind) and Yoga Nidra (sleep) should be maintained. Do not practice yoga merely by studying books, watching television or by watching others practice it. Beginners should first take lessons from a qualified and experienced Yoga expert. Pregnant women should avoid Yoga Asanas, Kapalbhati (Pranayamas), Bhastrika (Pranayamas) and Suryabhedana (alternate nostril breathing starting through right nostril).

Asanas could be practiced during pregnancy up to the first 80-90 days. Pranayama can be continued without Kumbhaka (breathing) throughout pregnancy, as it helps considerably during labour.

In general everyone should incorporate eating more raw food (salad and fruits). Drink at least 8-10 glasses of water every day. Reduce consumption of salt, sweets, spices and chilies. Avoid tea, coffee, fried food, smoking, alcohol, drugs and chewing tobacco.

Avoid other physical exercises like gymnastics, weightlifting, jogging, tennis, swimming etc for at least 20 minutes after asanas, pranayama and yoga.

Yoga is a way of life. It must be practised regularly and conscientiously, with thorough preparation, bearing all precautions in mind for true mental and physical relaxation. One has to also keep in mind that any results depend purely upon the individual, the nature of potential ailments and the regularity of the yogic practice.

It is here that Yoga comes to our assistance. Yoga emphasizes treatment of the root cause of any ailment. It works in a slow, subtle and miraculous manner. Modern medicine can claim to save a life at a critical stage, but, for complete recovery and regaining of normal health, one must rely on the efficacy of Yoga and Ayurveda. If there is a force that has created an ailment there is an equivalent opposite force that can heal it.

The Yogic way of life includes a code of ethics, regulations, discipline and much more, combined with meditation. Even a discussion of these subjects helps to relieve mental tensions and change attitudes. Simple Asanas help to stretch and relax the whole body and neutralize tensions. The consistent practice of yoga postures benefits all levels of our experience; from the restoration of balance, flexibility, poise, health and well being on a physical level to the cultivation of mental equanimity, emotional balance, and inner strength. On a body level Yoga postures stimulate and cleanse the glands, organs, muscles and nerves in ways that traditional exercise cannot.

Muscle tightness and strain is quickly relieved and both circulation and digestion improve. Stress-related symptoms like poor sleep, fatigue, muscle spasms, anxiety and indigestion are greatly improved.

Through continued practice Yoga postures can have a profound effect on the inner dimensions of life, establishing deep calm, concentration and emotional stability. Every human being is born with powers to make his or her life more meaningful and complete.

Physical power fulfills our physical needs through action; psychological power enables us to achieve the impossible in a modern world and our inner power helps us master the art of living by plugging us into infinite intelligence. Unfortunately, this inner power is the least utilized, and the lack thereof can lead to physical and psychological breakdowns.

Yoga is rooted in ancient history and helps to overcome physical and mental diseases by enhancing the cosmic power within us. Yoga is usually associated with yogis; as a method used at high altitudes to attain peace. However, it has no relevance to any particular religion.

It is a way of life to control and direct the mind, body and soul in the direction of attaining completeness.

The yogic system provides a path to the realization of our full human potential, rather than just mere improvements in our health, body and mind. Its true purpose is to expand our life to the fullness of our capacity. Life has provided us with 5 senses and with a consciousness. Our 5 senses are only geared towards our survival process, but in order to see further and beyond survival we need to develop and enhance our perception capabilities. The entire yoga system exists to bring about the enhancement of this perception. It is a system we can make use of to expand our awareness beyond our current limitations, beyond our confined thinking and beyond our physicality. We must finally realize that we are the only species on earth endowed with the intelligence that allows us to access that realm which is unseen, and come to the realization that who we are is inherently non physical even if it may not appear that way.

In order to help us in the process and depending on the capability of the person several types of yoga have been created such as Sahaj Yoga, Hatha Yoga, Raj Yoga, Kriya Yoga.

As we come to the greater understanding that we are intrinsically tied to the cosmos, we are looking to align our geometry with the geometry of the cosmos. Individuals who are able and enjoy training their body to achieve greater movement will gravitate towards hatha yoga. For those who want to go at a slower rhythm these individuals will prefer to practice kriya yoga and Sahaj yoga.

Any Yoga practice to help us attain enlightenment and liberation is recommended to be performed under the guidance of a capable Guru who can lead us through the deep aspects of Yoga like chanting, conceptualization and meditation. The idea that by merely performing Asanas (Postures) we can reach these elevated states of being is false and has been misleading to many. It is important to always keep in mind *that only the focused internal work combined with the practice of Asanas and Pranayamas will lead us there. When performed incorrectly there is always the possibility of hurting ourselves us complications may occur when we force our bodies to an extreme, specifically when holding the breath beyond our current capacity. Our capacity is known and defined by our Guru or teacher who also guides us in how and when to practice, guides our diet and also which herbs to take to optimize our body for yogic exercises.*

When we understand that Yoga is a way of life, there are two ways of going about it. We can incorporate it in our daily routine and continue being part of the world (this version is called Pravritti) or we can decide to detach from the world, by going into isolation (called Nivriti) and make the practice the main aspect of our everyday life. There is no difference between the two paths on a physical level. The difference only relates to our mental state of being and how detached we are from the worldly affairs. In the case of Pravritti we are still entangled with the world, in the case of Nivritti we remain a part of the world but we are not attached to it.

One of the wonders of the path of Yoga is that it helps to dissipate the ego, allowing our higher self to take over all levels of our being. In this process all our accumulated Karmas transform into so-called "devoted karmas". This allows us to rid ourselves of the possible consequences those karmas had us locked into. Let's begin by defining karma as any action, including anything involved in our daily routine. Every action generates a karmic re-action. Here we should clarify the difference between two different kinds of karmas. The first classification defines devoted and non devoted karmas. Devoted karmas are those performed by us but inspired by our higher self. In this state our identity has merged with Source and no ego is present in these actions. The second kind are non devoted karmas which are driven by our sense of our ego, where we have the perception of being responsible for them and deserving of merit. An example would be a person loans somebody money for them to pay their debt and improve their credit score, a non devoted karma person wants recognition for the higher credit score and better lifestyle this person now has, a devoted karma person knows they are just a channel through which Source flows energy of abundance into Earth. Now within non devoted karmas there is yet a subdivision: let's call them good and bad karmas. As we know the perception of good or bad has always been determined by society and has been instilled in us through our parents, the school system, law enforcement and religion, it is a way of controlling the masses. The concept of good and bad exists mainly to control humanity, by punishing the bad we instill fear and facilitate compliance. We have been trained to serve the purpose of groups in society rather than surrendering to the knowing of our higher self. Once we understand the dual nature of these karmas we are then called to inspired action from our inner being, our actions will be devoted, free of ego and its consequences. As long as we continue to live titillating within the boundaries of good and evil in a duality mindset, we will not break free from the consequences these karmas are generating, therefore making it difficult to attain higher self and ultimately liberation. Only once having evolved this aspect of our existence we move into alignment, and then even the smallest action turns into a meaningful one. A person who reaches the stillness and consciousness of living solely by devoted actions (karmas), has not even the slightest desire left to hurt another person, that alone would be life altering in the history of humanity.

Every action that we perform in our external experience is a consequence of our inner world, so the way we think and feel is crucial to the way we will live, perceive life and interact with others. We must cultivate our inner self with thoughts of unity, gratitude, appreciation and knowing that all is well. In addition we must engage in daily yogic practices that will generate in us the perfect environment for bliss to blossom. The more we come to terms with the oneness of our existence and are able to drop the duality mentality we will have learned to coexist with our ego in a way it can serve us. We will then raise the vibration of the ego or the self to resonate with the frequency of our higher self, that bright inner intelligence that beats in every one of our cells.

CHAPTERS OR LIMBS OF YOGA

1 YAMA (RESTRAINS) - ACTIONS WE SHOULD AVOID

This is the process of purifying our energy through our interaction with the world.

10 sublimbs:

1. *Non violence (Ahimsa),*
2. *Truth (Satya),*
3. *Non stealing (Asteya),*
4. *Celibacy (Brahmacharya)*
5. *Forgiveness and patience (Kshama),*
6. *Steadfastness (Dhriti)*
7. *Compassion (Daya),*
8. *Simplicity (Saralta),*
9. *Dietary Control (Mitahara),*
10. *Purity (Shauch) (outer and inner)*

Outer purity is done by Earth (soap and water) ; Neti (water cleaning through nostrils), Dhauti (cleaning of stomach with cloth) and Vasti (cleaning of intestines through enema).

Inner purity consists of the understanding that we are our soul and not our body; having purity of mind.

1. Ahimsa (Non-Violence)

Ahimsa is the yogic principle of non-violence which should be geared towards all living beings. Through this practice we arrive at a state of existence in which all life is seen and perceived as the self. By practicing non-violence we can step by step reach a stage in which we learn to experience ourselves through all other humans and all animals. How could you possibly harm that which you consider to be you or an extension of yourself. We then love everyone and everything equally, which gives us the awareness of not harming any being in any way, neither through words nor physical actions.

Ahimsa, if rightly understood, it is the ultimate tool to turn one's enemy into a friend, thereby avoiding conflict. Mahatma Gandhi used this tool to free India from the British rule and achieved what was considered an impossible task. Through the practice of non violence from a yoga perspective we understand that everything stems from the same source energy which flows equally through all beings. When we start loving all creatures in the universe as if they are our own self, respecting them as such, all conflicts tend to resolve completely.

The principle of Ahimsa is only successfully mastered when we manage to apply it even in the simplest of areas in our lives, not just in obvious and maybe extreme situations. It is to be understood that to harm another in the slightest way, even by disrespect, not only does it harm the person at the receiving end but it causes even more harm to the perpetrator. Mastery of Ahimsa therefore is very rare. Many people would not actually kill others but it is very common for most of us to anger each other, gossip, think badly of each other or glance at each other with negativity as all of this is violence. It is essentially our mindset, rather than our physical actions that can either lead us towards liberation, or hold us in greater bondage through suffering. Ahimsa is best described as an attitude of harmlessness and a demeanor of universal benevolence.

2. Satya (Truth)

"Asato Ma Sat Gamaya (From untruth towards truth") - Upanishads

"Truth is God and God is truth" - Mahatma Gandhi.

Truth is a very deep concept, it's purpose is to express who we really are and what we believe through our words, expressions and actions. Expressing our experiences in a sweet and soft manner is called "Truth". It is the second aspect of the Yama section and our work is to try to ponder every sentence before speaking.

Complete honesty with ourselves requires us to create a little bit of space between our thoughts and our words which requires stillness or at least some slowing-down of the mind. When we react instantly to situations on a purely compulsive and emotional level we often are not seeing the truth and are acting from a place of fear and conditioning. Once we realize that our true self is not composed of our thoughts and our emotions, we experience some inner relief, as we start to separate the illusion of who we think we are from who we really are; Our soul.

Truth is not merely limited to the words we speak, it also encompasses our actions and the way we portray ourselves (for example pretending and misleading someone to achieve our goals). We should always be true to our nature, our essence and be committed to the truth through our words, actions and most of all our intentions. This requires deep understanding, great awareness and dedication to honesty.

Truth is also deeply connected to who we are, in the deepest core of ourselves. In order to be in a state of being in which we are one with the truth we want to learn to be able to detach from our emotions. This way we can be conscious that our words have integrity and are in alignment with our authentic self. Honest communication, and living a life of integrity are the foundations for all relationships, not only the one with others and society as a whole but also with ourselves.

We have been led to believe that intuition stems from our higher self and that it always tells us the truth, when in reality our intuition is often based on an illusionary state. It is important to know that in the moment intuition strikes us, it will always be accompanied by a false message, therefore there is a chance for it to be unreliable. The best way to use our intuitive power is to be careful to always trust the very first thought that comes to our minds, which is usually the true aspect of our intuition. By relying on this first thought, we can better keep ourselves from acting on the illusory aspects that follow the first message.

Often in our lives when we are faced with emotional challenges which can make it difficult to be truthful, especially when we are in love or conflict. In such situations where conflict and fear can threaten us, it is easier to be tempted to be untruthful as we are trying to portray a specific self image that is not necessarily our true self. These are specifically the times when it is important to understand ourselves. These situations test us and open the opportunity to look deep inside ourselves before speaking up. If we find ourselves deviating from the truth, we should avoid speaking at all.

The key element before speaking is to pause and let your thought or the words we are about to speak be tested by the following three questions, if it does not pass one or more. Do not speak:

Is it true?
Is it necessary to speak?
Will it be kind to speak?

If your words are going to be considerate and gentle, go ahead and speak; Otherwise refrain. What is the goal? What are we trying to accomplish?

If we feel that someone has misbehaved towards us and our counterpart feels justified in their actions and words, we can politely talk to them and explain our viewpoint without being harsh and unkind in return. In any discussion what is right should be more important than who is right. The fact remains that our ego might not allow us to accept that the other person is entitled to have a different opinion to ours. We, at a social level, should respect others' opinions even if we do not agree with them. However we should not allow ourselves to get exploited because we want to be kind. It is possible to communicate with clarity and firmness and still do it in a gentle manner.

There are three types of truth in this world: absolute truth, relative truth and untruth. Absolute truth is equally understood and accepted by everyone. Untruth is also very clear therefore there are no disputes in that area. All conflict is centered around relative truths. For example, followers of any religion or politics believe that they hold the truth to the universe. Their belief itself isn't the issue. The problem arises when we think we are the only ones to hold the truth and others do not. Therefore the only solution is to develop tolerance towards all, to live in harmony with each other and not to impose our views on life onto others. This will allow us to equally work on our strengths and weaknesses with curiosity and kindness.

3. Asteya (Non stealing)

Non stealing on a superficial level obviously relates to abstaining from taking physical things that don't belong to us. The original and deeper concept behind it is that stealing can also be committed through our speech, our actions and even through our desires. Something as harmless as taking someone's time or talking to someone about a disturbing topic could be considered taking somebody's peace of mind. Therefore it relates to not taking that which has not been offered to us, including material things, time, thoughts, ideas, emotions, and energy. This view and way of life requires a deep level of consciousness.

We must never look for situations or anything at all outside of ourselves to make us happy and fulfilled. Happiness and fulfillment only come from within, they are inherently a part of us. Therefore the urge to steal always comes from an illusory place of fear, of lack, scarcity and sometimes even from greed. The task is to grab a handle on our views to avoid succumbing to these fear based dark holes. For all those seeking the path of a yogi it is a vital element to refrain from looking outside of themselves.

Asteya refers to the concept of honoring our body as well as our social and financial status, just as they are in the here and now. Even as we continue to push forward and work towards our goals and aspirations it is important to acknowledge that the universe is a vast and abundant place in which there is plenty for all of us to be, do or have anything we want. We must move away from the idea that this is a limited pie, and a scarcity mentality that by someone having something somehow it is taking it away from me. On the contrary it is a vast universe that continues to expand with the growth of human desire. The need to compare our situation to others will always lead us to inevitable suffering. What others possess should never be any of our concern as it will not serve us in a positive way. Therefore we are working to shift our mindset from lack and scarcity to abundance and satisfaction.

4.   Brahmacharya (Celibacy):

Celibacy is a voluntary vow of sexual abstinence. It is not connected to the religious sacrament of marriage. Initially in the old days, thousands of years ago, celibacy meant literally not to engage in any sexual activity; neither through our speech (talking about sex), nor though our heart's desire (thinking of sex) nor through sexual intercourse itself. However, as times progressed so did the understanding of sexual restraint. Sometimes it refers to abstaining from the act of intercourse, sometimes to being in a monogamous relationship with love and mutual respect without any outside sex.

There are other immensely valuable aspects related to sex that need to be considered when we engage with a sexual partner. We all have a physical body and an energy body which extends beyond our physical boundaries. Therefore, every intimate interaction also brings an energy exchange which happens predominantly through our energy field. This means that part of the other person's essence blends with our field and at the same time part of our field blends with the other person. Now how is this relevant to us? This energy exchange can have a disturbing effect on both parties involved. This happens because both energies try to balance themselves like it happens in the case of electricity. Energy will flow from higher to lower potential level, thereby depleting the person who has a higher energy charge in the interaction. This happens even in conversational interactions, but obviously during sexual intercourse a blending of the two fields is most prevalent. The other important aspect to mention is that this is not limited to "good energy" it also translates to "negative" and karmic energy. We will be vulnerable to absorb undesired energies, therefore, being very perceptive and conscious of our sexual mates is of major importance. If we were to have the capacity to divert this external energy and not have it disturb our own field, there would be no problem. But this can only be achieved at the stage of enlightenment. Until then we should try to avoid having multiple sex partners, or a partner that is with mutiple people in an effort to preserve our energy field from being affected.

Celibacy should also be practiced through our speech, intentions and actions. For example compulsive thoughts about sex should be avoided. But here lies the question: who wants to be celibate and what for? The answer is simple, it aids in the attainment of divine consciousness. You can be certain that by practicing this method of attaining connection to the divine we can effectively live an extraordinary life. This practice brings good health, inner strength, peace of mind, and long life. It also invigorates the mind and the nerves, helps to conserve physical and mental energy, it enhances our memory, willpower, and brain function. It restores strength, vigor and vitality. We will feel a shift in our overall health and wellbeing as strength and fortitude are obtained. Usually an individual who is successful in the practice of Brahmacharya will have a sweet voice, a beautiful complexion and lustrous eyes.

5. Kshama (Forgiveness)

The literal translation is forgiveness, however the quality to be developed and enhanced in the seeker of the yogic way is patience. If we do not possess this quality we will not be able to manifest forgiveness.

Kshama involves exercising patience, the restraint of intolerance towards others especially under difficult circumstances. One of the goals is to try to be as agreeable as possible. We should try to reach a level where we allow others to behave according to their nature, without needing them to adjust their behavior in any way to please us. Part of the re-learning process is to overcome the need to argue, the need to dominate conversations or interrupt others. An important aspect is to maintain a calm demeanor and avoid being in a hurry. We should be of a patient heart with children and the elderly likewise.

We should always try to minimize inner stress within us by keeping our worries at bay, making an effort to remain poised in good as well as bad times.

Forgiveness is the result of a patient inner atmosphere. It is not something we seek to do, it is something that happens when our inner foundation allows for it.

An individual who is inherently impatient is a reflection of unfulfilled desires. It is important to notice when we seem to have no time (patience) for interruptions or delays from anything that might seem irrelevant to what we are trying to achieve. If we are observant we will notice that after some time this impatience of ours will become frustration. The question is, how do we go about overcoming this unwanted state of mind? The solution is to focus on living in the eternity of the present moment. Living in the present moment creates an internal atmosphere within us in which we feel complete. We feel like we have nothing further to achieve or accomplish because all is provided for and no past or future can change that.

The magic lies in the power of acceptance, which means accepting people around us and accepting life events just the way they are. This attitude has the power to eliminate impatience and intolerance from us completely.

In order to develop this kind of acceptance within us we must be aware of the law of karma and we should remind ourselves that source is in all things, in all people, at all times. We must come to terms with what is, thereby accepting the perfection of divine timing in the creation, the preservation and expansion of the universe. When I say preservation I mean be at peace with the fact that there has never been a time when the universe has not existed, yes that is right -there is no beginning nor will there ever be an end to its constant expansion.

The beauty of understanding the law of karma is that it provides peace of mind, allowing us to understand that everything taking place is divinely guided by Source. The moment this concept registers inside our soul, we are able to accept that no external occurrence has really anything to do with us. It's in this beautiful moment when the veil is lifted and our ego dissolves completely, that acceptance has now become a part of us.

6. Dhriti (Steadfastness)

What does it mean to foster steadfastness? It is the art of overcoming fear and indecision. We must know that we are able to have it all, if the universe has granted us the capacity to dream it, it has also provided us the capabilities to have it. We can achieve our desires through prayer, purpose, plan, persistence and push. It is paramount to always remember to be firm in our decisions, and to avoid sloth and procrastination at all costs. It is of crucial importance to develop willpower and courage. We should always keep in mind that in order to overcome obstacles it is best to never carp or complain. If we are convinced of our goal we should never let opposition or fear of failure result in changing our direction. Never drink the poison of doubt and fear.

The meaning of Dhriti is to act with determination and fortitude.

That means the determination present in humans that makes us strive continuously towards our desired goal which will provide us with courage, enthusiasm and perseverance to face and overcome all obstacles in our way.

Consistency is the key to the conquest of karma, and also the key to progress on our spiritual path, a clear purpose and plan is needed before persistence will have any effect. But in order to succeed under any circumstance it is of utmost importance that I have certainty and faith in my success, a kind of faith that never wavers.

There must be a constant light within us, that shines at all times to lead the way on our path, a light that doesn't flicker and never forsakes us. For there is NO doubt in me "I will succeed". I am firm in my thought, and I know without a shadow of a doubt that nothing can come between me and my desire. It is law, it can be no other way.

7. Daya (Compassion)

A person on the yogic path will strive to practice compassion. But what is compassion, and what does it entail? It means to conquer all callous, cruel and insensitive feelings towards all beings. It is the ability to see God everywhere and in all things. It is the result of being kind to people, animals, all plants and the Earth itself. It involves forgiving those who apologize and show true remorse, while not holding on to unnecessary grudges. It goes hand in hand with fostering sympathy for others in need who might be going through any type of suffering or struggle. It means honoring and assisting those who are weak, impoverished, aged or in pain. As a result we will also automatically oppose any type of family abuse and other cruelties.

Through it we give clemency, absolution and forgiveness even to the most hideous mistakes. When someone has done wrong by us, we will want to look the other way and be compassionate. It will elevate us by transcending resentment to a degree that will even make us care for the suffering of someone who has wronged us.

Compassion is the consequence of love.

And what is love?

Love is the outgrowth of understanding and understanding is outgrowth of reason.

Daya is all encompassing, it involves the biggest acts of kindness and the smallest ones as well.

It will require true will and determination to evolve on this path as it is spiritually very advanced to achieve this quality. It entails having awareness and deep understanding towards everyone, in every situation. We will learn to grasp the truth about being in a state of bliss and grow as a consequence of it.

8. Arjava (Honesty)

How do we maintain honesty? This question has an easy answer. We achieve it by renouncing any sort of deception and wrongdoing. The task here is to act honorably even when going through hard times. This includes being lawful, paying our taxes, being straightforward in business and simply doing an honest day's work. When following this path it would be out of the question to ever consider bribing or accepting a bribe. It is of monumental importance not to ever cheat anyone or on anyone, deceive or circumvent anyone to achieve an end. The goal is to always be frank with ourselves. Facing and accepting our own faults is without a doubt vital when on this path; never blaming others for our shortcomings and to know the only truth is that we are the creators of our own reality.

In order to move forward on our yogic path we should strive to always be honest with ourselves, confront our problems face on, admit that we carry all the responsibility for them and make soulful decisions towards solving them.

It is often the frustrated and discontent people who are not honest with themselves as they blame others for their own faults and predicaments. They always look for scapegoats to blame to avoid accountability.

Honesty begins in our own heart and soul and once it is anchored inside of us it will radiate outward into the world, when we interact with others. A very visual way of noticing when we are in the midst of blaming others, is by acknowledging that the moment you point your index finger at someone, the remaining three fingers are pointing back at you. This indicates to us where the responsibility lies. The main quality to be developed is straightforwardness with our life partner, with our children, with our family, our neighbors and our government.

Our aim is to be: non manipulative, go the extra mile, be nice and accept others the way they are, not have critical thoughts and don't try to change anyone.

9.   Mitahara (Moderate Appetite)

I think we underestimate the importance that food plays in our spiritual development. Also on the yogic path it is imperative to be moderate in our food intake, the number one dietary measure to increase longevity is food restriction. The idea is to be conscious about the amount of food we consume. We should try to reduce or eliminate foods like meat, fish, shellfish, fowl or eggs, there should be no greater joy than to choose fresh, wholesome vegetarian foods that revitalize our bodies.

There are 3 types of food: positive, negative and neutral pranic food. Let's start by explaining positive pranic food; it uplifts and enhances our energy level, this type gets digested quickly and does not rot in our system (fruits, vegetables, nuts, sprouted seeds). Then we have negative pranic foods which are all those with an addictive quality and that stimulate our nervous system, they tend to give our system a boost of energy only to withdraw the energy from the body thereafter (garlic, chili, coffee, tea, intoxicants, marihuana, junk food and processed food). Lastly we have neutral pranic food which increases lethargy in our system and laziness, they tend to increase our desire to sleep (potatoes and tomatoes are main ones, and should be avoided by those with arthritis and joint issues). The suggestion is to avoid negative pranic food at all costs, drink in moderation, try to eat at regular times, and don't eat between meals. Always respect your body, don't refuel when the tank is overflowing. It is vital that meals always are taken in a peaceful atmosphere and that we eat at a moderate pace.

All foods contain energy, all energy comes from the sun. Therefore it is advisable that a yogi's lifestyle will follow a simple diet. The first and best type of energy source would be to get it directly and only from the sun. This seems impossible but some have achieved it. The second best way to source our energy is through food whose energy has come directly from the sun like fruits and vegetables. The third best source to get our energy is from animals which themselves had as their diet those sun energized vegetables like cows, sheep and others. The fourth and last would be from animals that have eaten other animals such as dogs who eat meat, cats, sharks, lions, etc.

Concerning our dietary habits there is a golden rule which states "less is more", it is important to eat in such a way where 1/4 of our stomach is filled with liquid, 1/2 with food and the other 1/4 remain available for air and digestive processes.

It is advisable to adhere to the following guidelines when it comes to the quantity of food intake. There is a simple rule of thumb. Amount of food per indidual depending upon the work they perform and is subdivided as follows per meal: spiritual people should only eat around 8 spoonfuls, a normal family person should eat no more than 32 spoonfuls, a single person 16 spoonfuls, a celibate can digest anything so there is no amount suggested and a sick person should try to eat as little as possible. Just keep in mind, there is nothing (other than drugs and smoking) that hurts the body more than excessive eating, both in terms of the amount of food as well as the quality of food. Anyone who eats rich, processed, dead food is not following mitahara and is effectively poisoning themselves.

10. Shaucha (Purity)

We can uphold the ethic of purity by avoiding impurity in our mind, body and speech. We can start by maintaining a clean, pure, uncluttered home and workplace. A yogi will always act virtuously, will want to keep good company, never mixing with adulterers, thieves and other impure people. A yogi will never be driven to engage in any type of violence nor ever use harsh, angered or indecent language. It will be part of our daily practice to meditate and keep ourselves in a peaceful state of being.

Part of the practice here involves being able to humbly express our remorse for any wrongdoing caused by us, acknowledge our mistake and willingly make amends to heal the situation. It means to sincerely apologize to those on the receiving end of our hurtful words and/or our actions. A yogi will always resolve all contention before going to sleep, will seek out and correct any faults or bad habits as it will be wise to welcome correction as a means to bettering ourselves. A yogi does not boast, nor show pride or pretension.

We are ultimately trying to achieve clarity, purity of mind, body and speech. All of these elements are essential for our health and wellbeing. The purity of our body is achieved by cleaning ourselves with water and earth (called soap). Purity of the mind is achieved by consciously choosing loving and pleasant thoughts that will keep us in a state of ease, any thought that is aligned with our inner being will always make us feel good. It is important to realize that we play a vital role when it comes to our happiness, as we are in control of what we choose to think and feel. The source of the "impurity" of our minds and the misery of mankind lies in the feelings of anger, hate, greed, pride, fear, and negative thoughts.

We will quickly realize that by consciously choosing more positive feeling thoughts and words, we reach a better state of emotion, therefore our vibration raises, and we achieve a higher state of consciousness. It is not a massive undertaking and can be easily attained through self observation with the goal to discover ourselves as the higher self we truly are. The key element is to care about how we feel. Our emotions are the alarm that gets set off when we are off course. Our only task is to get out of our own way by relaxing, and knowing that the greater part of us is our non physical self who is ever present and always guiding the way. When we are in complete alignment we are worry-free, joyful and at ease. Our emotions are our biggest asset, if we use them as our compass to show us where we are at any given time in relationship to our real self. Every time we feel lousy, shameful, unworthy and afraid it's just evidence that we are out of sync. When we feel anything other than joy, that discord is the way we have of knowing we need to make our way back to the self, and this can be achieved through meditation and mindfulness.

The body can be purified through shatkarma yoga which removes toxins and involves the following procedures:

Netī is what we call a nasal wash. This is the practice of cleaning and purifying our breathing system through two different methods, we can use either. The first being jal neti by using a neti pot to cleanse the nasal passages. We insert water through one nostril, tilt the head and the water pours out the other nostril, and we repeat the procedure through alternating nostrils. A basic neti wash consists of purified water and non-iodized salt, to create a gentle saline solution. It can also be performed with a set of threads called sutra neti which is done by inserting thread through one nostril, when it touches the tongue you pull it out through the mouth, and then repeat the alternate nostril. The benefit is a complete cleanse of nasal cavity from any accumulated impurities and therefore no hindrance of prana energy flow into the system through our breathing.

Dhautī is the cleansing of the whole digestive tract. It mainly consists of cleaning the food pipe either with warm water in the morning or through inserting a piece of cloth which we will swallow and then pull back out to clean the food passage from accumulation just as you would do with any plumbing pipe at home. You can also perform it through vamana dhauti, which is mainly by drinking a large amount of salted warm water and then vomiting it out to remove all extra mucus and other remaining particles of food that built up onto the food pipe, this is also called Kunjal Kriya.

Naulī is a self-administered abdominal massage, which we do by only contracting the abdominal wall muscles. Thereby we stand with the feet about hip width apart, hands on knees, and body at about a 45 degree angle. The core is rotated internally by moving the abdominal muscles alternately in a clockwise, then in a counterclockwise direction.

Basti is a colonic irrigation commonly known as enema. It can be water enema or coffee enema. It is simply to insert 500 ml of warm water through the anus and retain it inside the large intestine for a period of 15-20 min and then release it along with all toxins that will be expelled through this process. In the period of time of withholding the water, it is advisable to churn the abdominal muscles to help detach impurities more effectively. In the case of the coffee enema you have the added benefit of releasing all the bile accumulated in the gallbladder tubes.

Kapālabhātī in Sanskrit means skull polishing, and is a pranayama breathing technique. This practice is intended to improve the function of our brain, and energize the chakra system by balancing our nadis (refer to Pranayama chapter). In the normal breathing our emphasis is on the inhale, whereas here the emphasis is on the exhale. When we emphasize more on the exhale, more impurities are released along with the carbon dioxide on our exhale. It is a sharp, short exhale followed by the relaxation of our core.

Trātaka is an eye exercise, where we focus steadily and continuously the direction of the gaze at a fixed point such as a black spot, a candle flame, rising sun or on our third eye chakra. When we focus on outer objects it is called outer trataka, and when we focus on our third eye it is *called inner trataka. The benefits include increase of brain concentration and purification of the mind from fluctuating thoughts.*

We have mentioned all the basic requirements needed to have a complete Shaucha practice, nonetheless please start under the guidance of a knowledgeable teacher. It is advisable to do some or all of these rituals on a regular basis, but not daily. The time frame between them should be about 3 months apart to not over tax our system. Also of great importance is to use sterile and clean products every time, and to follow mitahara (diet control) rigorously during the processes. Be in a pleasant state of being when involved in any of the above mentioned.

There are several benefits to practicing Shaucha, some of them include internal purification that enhance the overall functioning of our external organs, balances all the elements in our system (earth, fire and water), channeling the flow of prana through the nadis (nerve system), reduces the likelihood of blockages in the system, helps the body-mind connection, enhances immune system, and reverses aging process.

2 NIYAMA (OBSERVANCES) - ACTIONS WE SHOULD ENGAGE IN

This is the process of purifying our internal energy, meaning through our thoughts and emotions.

10 sublimbs:

1. Tapas (Perseverance),
2. Santosha (Contentment),
3. Aastikata (Believer),
4. Daan (Donation),
5. Ishwar Puja (Worship),
6. Shraavak (Adhering to the Natural Principles),
7. Hri (Managing shame),
8. Mati (Desire to attain self),
9. Japa (Chanting),
10. Vrat aur Hut (Fasting and fire rituals).

1. Tapas (Perseverance)

Before anything else in our life we should strive to develop perseverance, it's the art of powering through anything with determination and focus, overcoming any obstacle and reaching our goals. And how is this concept any different from Dhriti explained in the "Yamas, Chapter 1"? In Dhriti we were explaining the actions to avoid "what not to do", *here we are focusing on what we must do. What actions do we need to engage in, to attain our desired outcome?*

First we need to fully comprehend that the circumstances the universe presents us with are always perfect. We need to accept them joyfully, trust and continue our path in pursuit of our goals. Never allow doubt have its way with us nor deviate us from the path we have chosen. All is well at all times, even when it looks tough. Our job is to move forward with a happy heart, even in the face of adversity, we must always know, this too shall pass. We call it in Sanskrit Dradhata, which literally means persist.

Anything we want to achieve in life requires determination; it takes perseverance to reach our life's purpose,

Here we will outline what to do in order to walk this path.

A mindset of "I will succeed" should be our life mantra. We also need faith and conviction that universal forces are always on our side when we are aligned with our inner knowing.

We need to keep on until we achieve the desired goal. How do we go about this? We persist when faced with life challenges no matter how difficult the challenge, we push forward and never deviate from our path or lose sight of our goal. Possible examples could be: persist in attaining someone's love no matter what, or to achieve a work position, to get pregnant, or to heal from a health condition. We can apply this to any arena in our life. The goal is to achieve continuance in a state of grace (never to feel bad or defeated) until our success is attained, this is vital.

Tapas in sanskrit also meant that in the old days people would go into the forest to practice their prayers until their desired results were achieved. It's an urgent effort directed towards a defined purpose. It's fulfilment is realized through discipline and self control, through a conscious and sustained effort to reduce all temptations and to overcome all obstacles. By self control I mean not to indulge in anything that might make us deviate from our goal. No difficulty or achievement should be an excuse or reason to deter us from our set path.

Tapas in yoga can be achieved through our body, speech and mind. Tapas of the body may use some of the yama practices like: celibacy, non violence and fasting. Tapas of the speech is known in sanskrit as mauna which is to live in silence for a certain period of time during the day. The highest mauna by far is mental silence. It is extremely beneficial in conserving our energy and sharpening our mind. Tapas of the mind signifies to have perfect peace of mind and automatic effortless self control. When we reach this state we are imbued with positive thoughts void of any pessimism. It has everything to do with our will power. It means perseverance in our daily actions, thoughts, emotions and practices. People who like practicing yoga have great enthusiasm in the initial phase but then the moment they encounter some lethargy they tend to quit. If we are persistent, our positive attitude will prevent us from faltering until we are a successful yogi. We will not feel any mental discomfort and we will consciously keep our mind and body at ease and in a blissful state.

2.   Santosha (Contentment)

The second is contentment which is known in Sanskrit as Santosha. It entails making a living in an honorable way by maintaining proper social standards and learning to be content and grateful with our achievements. It doesn't mean that we do not want growth and expansion for our business but rather not to be greedy and unhappy with our current situation. Whatever the circumstance is in the present moment: expansion or absence of it. Santosha is the ability to always foster happiness in our heart regardless of the situation.

Santosha is about joyfully accepting without uselessly spending energy on living in the past nor fantasizing about the grand future. As both are a misuse of the privileged faculty we have as humans to remember and project into the future, and a complete waste of our time.

There is a big difference between setting a goal with a clear vision and fantasizing about what we would like to change. A goal is concrete and focused while fantasizing does not help us reach our objective, it is just unhappiness with what is.

To accept and love the world as it is, is considered contentment. It can also be described as an attitude in which we don't have the desire to change anything in the world other than disturbance in our thought patterns. We come to the understanding that we only need to change ourselves. This is achieved by calibrating our internal chemistry, yes you heard it right. We are the largest and most efficient pharmaceutical factory on earth, we have the ability to produce any hormone at will. It can be serotonin which makes us happy or cortisol and adrenaline which stress our system. This is entirely up to us and completely in our control. We learn to only focus on our inner capabilities to improve ourselves and as a consequence everything in our surroundings is seen through a new set of eyes.

Santosha is focusing on the present moment and living fully, with complete absence of negativity. It is acknowledging the uniqueness in every moment. Whatever life has provided us with we will accept willingly and with a happy heart. When we are in a state of being where we are not trying to change anyone or any circumstance around us, we allow for everything we desire to make its way to us as we are no longer a resisting force working against it.

3. Aastikata (Believer)

The third is the believer aspect of our soul. We abide by our faith, convictions and beliefs and therefore we are not followers of the beliefs and convictions of other people or institutions (as in the case of religion). In Aastikata our beliefs are born from within us and we live by them.

This involves faith in our true self, belief in God, and conviction in our source energy.

When we refer to God here we speak of our higher self, the source of all creation. Through the science of yoga we can deepen the study of the inner self which ultimately leads to the discovery of our higher self.

Progress happens mostly through self contemplation, meaning that the self awareness, wisdom and knowing will come to us by looking at ourselves more closely via meditation and reaching self awareness.

4. Daan (Donation)

Fourth is the aspect of donation whereby we share a portion of all our earnings with society. A minimum of one tenth of our earnings is to be put aside for our spiritual teachers or the needy.

It is considered charity to share in reverence with those who have given us wisdom. It is important that this sharing comes from legal earnings. This is how it has been said by Shiva who was the first yogi who ever lived. It is customary for these donations to be given in the form of actions, words, religious books, food, praise in your heart, time or in any other form. The best donation is one where we go out of your way and physically visit the needy and give it directly without making them feel that we are trying to help them. The second best way is to invite the person to our place and offer what we want to share in person. In either case the goal is to share without the ego of giving. When the ego of giving is out of the picture we don't expect anything in return.

There is much beauty in sneaking in a donation like Santa Claus without anyone noticing. It is a beautiful Nyama and it keeps the spiritual energy of unity running throughout us as we see only one life. We can share anything from clothes to books for children, to donating our time in any type of institution. Our knowledge and education is a great gift to share when we practice this observance.

The moment we expect something in return, the concept of donation goes out the window and it becomes a transaction. Our sharing no longer retains its purity, as our intention is not pure. We must also be vigilant in not promoting beggary, or pity money by giving "charity" in the street. We must see others as source sees them, as light and in full potential of attaining anything they desire when they are in alignment. Every human is equally capable, no one is more or less connected to Source. Our attention should never be in noticing lack in anyone, by giving pity money we increase the energy of scarcity in the receiver instead of reducing it, it enhances it hence rendering the act counterproductive.

There is also the concept of sharing with uninvited guests (atiti in sanskrit). This is also considered a donation, given you had intended for that meal or whatever to be for you and now you have chosen to share it with someone unexpectedly. We are to treat our guests in a godly way in this context.

All those who cannot donate money or anything tangible are always capable of donating their wisdom. We can share our talent and time without seeking praise.

5.   Ishwar Puja (Worship)

Fifth is related to Worship, it means to be in a state of permanent communication with source and to totally surrender to the cosmic will. We surrender our mind and body completely, absolutely and thoroughly to the cosmic forces. Therefore all our goals can be achieved when we are consciously cooperating with life. Through devotion and sincerity we blend with universal harmony and we gain access to the higher frequency of the cosmos.

The term we use in Sanskrit is Ishwar puja. It refers once more to having a happy mind and a joyous heart, a sort of undeniable faith and living by truth. It involves the unification of the feminine and masculine universal forces. Recognizing this aspect of life and always paying respect to this energy is vital. The happiness that comes from achieving a certain *level of unification of the feminine and masculine energies in our heart is in and of itself considered worship.*

The best practice for this observance is to cultivate devotion through daily meditation, that is effectively the way our soul evolves from the time of its conception to its return to source. The purpose of our existence is the joyous expansion of our soul in a journey that titilates from darkness to light as we uncover our preferences along the way, finally reaching liberation from our identity. At some point the desire for liberation sparks within us; then we become driven by the positive qualities that live within the seven chakras which are: strength, pleasure, will power, love, communication, intuition and connection to source.

Our physical self is made of 5 elements namely earth (food), water, fire, air and space (or nothingness also known as the divine).

Meanwhile our higher self consists of only 3 elements: air, fire and space. Therefore our higher self can neither accept food nor water directly. How does this matter to us, and what is the relevance here? It can help us understand the importance of fire rituals and how in many traditions fire bridges the connection between the physical and the divine. This happens through the use of either candles, incense, or bonfire. Whenever humans want to connect to their higher self through an offering, usually it is done with the help of the fire element. Let me give you a simple explanation: If I give you a banana and you eat it, can you give it back to me? The answer is no. And even if I was to get it back after you ate it, would I be able to consume it? The answer is NO. In the same way, when we give an offering to our higher self we should not be able to take back what has been offered. Therefore all offerings are done through fire as it consumes it and blends it to the nothingness that is Source. It's considered auspicious and we are able to attain the power of nature through it.

The concept of offering in the yogic traditions refers to receiving a blessing. When we want to receive something from our higher self, we use worship and rituals to connect.

Once we are liberated and reach a higher level of consciousness, all our desires die off and at this stage we become one with our higher self, leaving behind any need for worship or rituals.

6.   Shraavak (Adhering to Natural Principles)

Sixth is Shraavak, this entails the capacity to follow or adhere to the wisdom instilled in us by our guru or sage. There is much we need to know about the natural principles present in the universe. We are encouraged to listen to a sage or guru, and let them guide us in the understanding of the cosmic forces and the innate wisdom that is responsible for all life.

The practice involves reading, studying and receiving the wisdom from those who understand the subtle lines between the forms of illusion we are entangled in. It is about truly embodying the wisdom imparted versus just listening to information.

What does it take to truly integrate this teaching? The only necessary quality is to be connected to a spiritual guide (the knower) and remain receptive to the energies transmitted which are beyond words and can be experienced only through meditative practices. It helps to meditate in the presence of our guru, be it in person or even at a distance, as time and space does not exist.

Siddhant means wisdom, principle of wisdom and the act of adhering to principles of wisdom.

The main requirement is to make ourselves as empty as possible before going to see a guru. Consider ourselves as a vessel. If the vessel is empty, it can be filled with universal truth. The path demands that we undo whatever past we have identified with, while knowing that our identity is purely cosmic. We can gain this knowledge by meditating, as it is a process of consciously deciding to quiet our mind and receive the impulses. Never seek a sage or guru in a state of desperation or sickness as they will not be able to make anyone their disciple or initiate a person under vulnerable circumstances.

We must seek a sage or guru with love in our heart, empty from past beliefs and void of doubt, this allows for our vessel to be filled with all the wonders and wisdom of the universe.

7.   Hri (Remorse or Management of Shame)

Seventh relates to shame or the seed of shame otherwise known as Hri in Sanskrit. But what is shame? It refers to the remorse we experience when we do something we perceive as wrong or when we fail to do something we feel we should have done. It is the feeling we experience each time we do something improper, something that embarrasses us.

The feeling of remorse is associated with feeling meek or inadequate in some way, shape or form. Sometimes it relates to the feeling of adversity we feel when we engage in activities frowned upon by Vedas (universal wisdom). Vedas are universal vibrations of wisdom present in the universe and those on the path of spirituality match this frequency and receive all the wisdom needed.

We are looking to attain a state of "shamelessness", when the result of our actions no longer matters to us. Having attained a shameless state means we have let go of our past and our present self image. It means we are able to resolve all our inner conflicts each night before going to sleep and wake up completely free each morning. It also means when we see faults and bad habits within us we can easily correct them, almost automatically.

Feeling shame is a common human experience which most of us are familiar with. We have to remember that even in the midst of experiencing these feelings, we can just as well let go and practice the art of disengaging. It is pointless and useless to harbor these feelings that hamper our spiritual growth. When it invades us, we tend to leave whatever we were pursuing in every aspect of life, and we risk losing it all.

Hri is that state in which nothing matters to us. Our past is of zero relevance to us, we shun pride, we don't feel pretension and we live in a state of being blissed out. We should make a conscious effort to welcome any correction as a means to better ourselves. When I say correction I mean we should accept our past as it was, never feel ashamed of it and to have the awareness moving forward to never do or say anything that would embarrass us. Hri or remorse is the most misunderstood observance or Niyama and it is definitely the most difficult to correct, humans never want to accept any wrongdoing. The more you point out to anyone what they have done wrong, the more they will defend and justify the reason for having done it. There is a real lack of role models in this department, the only one that comes to mind is Mahatma Gandhi who openly wrote a book revealing to the world everything he had done in his past and how he would never fall in those steps again.

When we have reached this state, we have learned to be at peace with all our decisions, we have understood the full meaning of what it means to refrain from non virtuous actions, and we have grown to recognize our mistakes on a deeper level. We are honest, we have finally surrendered our "self". Thereby we have reached a state that allows us to abandon feelings of shame rooted in our perceived inadequacies. In this state shame ceases to exist since that unnecessary fuel has been removed from our being.

8. Mati (Desire to Attain Self)

Eight is the desire to attain self otherwise known as Mati in Sanskrit. We can define this aspect as the state of desire-lessness, which we have achieved when we no longer seek worldly pleasures. Once we have overcome the passionate (irresistible, obsessive, compulsive) desires of the mind, we can now face all criticism with courage. Once we have silenced the illusory games of the mind, we have mastered the Nyama of Mati.

The consciousness of Mati is obtained by letting go of greed, possessiveness and attachment. Attempting to attain it brings up the question of our imagination and its usefulness. "Imagining" refers to the things we dream of, the mental pictures we paint of the things we want. The only time we "imagine" is when we desire something. Letting ourselves fall into our imagination leads to greed as we always want to possess what we are dreaming up (may this be a great marriage, good health, material objects, etc....). As we move closer to Mati we will encounter a catch twenty-two. In the beginning we need to want Mati to start moving into its direction but then at some point we will have to let go of even wanting to reach there. Once we integrated the conundrum of getting there by not wanting to get there, we will have overcome a major hurdle in the process of integrating the thought intelligence of Mati.

We must let go of it all, we must relinquish the search for worldly pleasures and focus all our attention on becoming one with source. In order to achieve this we must set aside all other thoughts. Most likely we will face criticism by others as they will perceive us as uninspired.

Once we have reached this higher level of awakening, we will be looking through our heart chakra and right through the veil of illusion, beyond the values of good and evil, which we previously had attached to all our interactions. We will have moved beyond, into a state of dissolution of matter.

Mati is the state of ultimate intelligence, in which we acquire desire-less-ness and put our mind into a state of total stillness in which there is no difference between criticism and praise. Opposites no longer carry any emotional meaning for us.

9. Jap (Chanting)

Ninth involves the act of chanting known as Japa in Sanskrit. Ja means to "destroy" and Pa means "sins", therefore chanting mantras has the ability to eliminate the karmas of birth, death and reincarnation.

Mantras are an exquisitely powerful tool as they hold the key to change and correct any circumstance in life. There is great strength to be found In chanting, it is most effective when given a specific mantra by a Guru and done regularly.

There are three types of chanting: Vaikharie, Upanshu and Manas. Vaikharie refers to speaking or singing the mantra out loud. Upanshu is the kind of chanting when our lips move but we make no sounds. In Manas everything happens inside our heart and not even our lips are moving. Upanshu is a thousand times more powerful than Vaikharie and Manas is again a thousand times more powerful than Upanshu.

Why does chanting mantras work? Based on the premise that the universe is in constant reverberation even if we are not aware of it, all creation began from sound. We then need to understand that the universe was created through the vibration of sounds and that all sounds emanate from A_U_M which created OHM. How is sound created? Consonants emanate masculine energy and vowels contain feminine energy. Each time consonants and vowels merge it is the unification of feminine and masculine energy therefore life is created as a consequence. By chanting we are blending with sounds that create a resonance within us to receive direct energy from source. It is a doorway to the universe. Through a continuous practice this energy starts to build up and gets stored within our chakras. From there we can redirect this energy towards any given purpose depending on our Sankalpa (intentions for what we wish to achieve). By applying this wisdom we transcend worldly happiness and gain access to ultimate happiness, and now can become one with all there is.

Jappa is not the mere repetition of words as there is no meaning in them, it is the contemplation and focus on a vibration that opens up a doorway, from there we simply stay on course with our original intention. We must control our scattered mind, and focus on these sounds so that they can become part of us. As explained above there are three types of chanting, and there also is the written version which is called Likhita.

The goal of chanting may greatly vary and can be used for material as well as spiritual gains. We should however focus only on one kind of goal to allow for the created energy to be contained until our desired goal is achieved. The actual mantra also varies greatly among different practitioners of Japa. Our Guru receives our individual mantra during the time of our initiation and then whispers it in our ear, only for us to hear.

A personal mantra needs to be individually received from source by a Guru and the student needs to be aware of its energy (each person has a specific dominant energy within them). A Guru is someone who has the ability to imbue students with the highest aspect of the mantra thereby anchoring them to Source. When a guru intentionally imbues us with the specific mantra energy, it works as a compass, connecting us directly to the energy of bliss each time we chant it. Mantras come with a stated goal of devotion, which can be liberation, enlightenment or maybe communicating with the divine. It is important to understand that mantras work most powerfully when they are activated with a particular intention and transferred to the student by a sage or guru at the time of initiation. Mantras can work even without initiation by a Guru. If we simply repeat known Mantras like "Ohm Namah Shiva" we will experience benefits like enjoyment and pleasure, but they will not help us if we are seeking enlightenment or a specific outcome as they do not offer the same transfer of energy.

10. *Vrata and Huta (Fasting and Fire Rituals):*

Tenth and final would be Huta and Vrata (Fire rituals and fasting) which occur under the guidance of a guru during the process prior, during and post initiation. Only after being initiated will your guru give a personal mantra and order a possible fasting (which can be anything: chanting, lack of eating, etc).

Huta is a ritual where an offering is required, it is also called a sacrifice ritual because the fire consumes our offering and thereby allows it to merge with source, thus we see it as a "sacrifice" or gift.

In the process of huta, we use fire as the agent and symbolic physical materials such as grains, clarified butter, milk and seeds as the offering. These material agents are symbolic of our anger, ego, fear, shame and hatred which are precisely what we are offering to be consumed or sacrificed in the fire. This ritual of using the element of fire to connect to source is also being used in many other establishments such as Christian churches in the form of candles, and in yoga centers, in various religious spaces, in Buddhism in the form of incense.

Our higher self or Source will contain these 3 elements: space, air and fire, therefore all religions practice their prayers in its presence. It can be in the form of candles, wax, incense sticks, etc. No ritual known as prayer will be performed in the absence of fire as it will carry no great value.

As we evolve on our spiritual path we attain a certain level of awareness where we are in tune with these elements present in us, as we are made up of earth, water, air, fire and space. When we come to the understanding that all these panchabhuta (earth, water, air, fire and space) are present in us and we can offer them from within us, we then no longer have the need for a fire ritual. We have reached a state of conscious awareness that I am not my body, thoughts or emotions, I am simply Source energy.

Rituals therefore are for those still on the path towards liberation who still identify with the physical aspect of their being and have not yet fully internalized the fact that our essence and source are the same.

The key when we perform these rituals in yoga is that we must perform a spiritual sacrifice along with it like letting go of our fear and all negative emotions including our ego.

Vrata relates to a vow, a resolve or devotion such as fasting, where we leave food and drinks aside for a while during the time frame we are performing our rituals and prayers. We may be seeking divine intervention for a healthy body, long life, serenity, fertility and/or happiness for ourselves and our loved ones, regardless what our motivation is initially, we stay committed and trust the process. The outcome depends on our level of trust, faith, inner strength and the belief that all blessings are achievable, knowing everything in this universe is working out for us. We must keep this resolve and level of commitment to ourselves during good and trying times equally, no matter how daunting the situation might seem.

What could we say to a person who is going through a very challenging time and has no more inner strength to carry on? We would say without hesitation to never give up, to know that once we are able to shift our mindset to see things in a different light and have a positive resolve about the circumstance we will gain the clarity and strength to achieve our goal.

When we find it difficult to meditate due to worry therefore we are unable to focus on our objective, or we have lost hope and feel depressed, we can look for support from our guru or spiritual teacher through energy transfer rituals. This connection can be done in person or at a distance and the energy gained in the process will help us reach our goals and objectives. (see additional chapter with results from case studies)

As a rule, there are five solutions to every problem we encounter in this universe. This realization will help us maintain a positive frame of mind - no matter what adversity we are facing it will reveal to us the answers we seek.

Some vratas are performed on a specific phase of the moon or during a certain planetary constellation. These auspicious times allow us to gain inner strength by tapping into an abundance of positive energy. Some of these occassions are full moon, new moon, the eleventh day of the moon, no moon and eclipses.

Vratas are usually of 3 types: kaika vrata is a vrata pertaining to our body where the focus is on physical austerity like fasting. In this case fasting can be done without drinking water called nirjala. Second is vachaika vrata pertaining to our speech and it is performed by abstaining from speaking, remaining in silent yoga for the desired period. The practitioner may drink water but may not eat solid food. And third is *manas vrata which entails controlling the mind of passions, or prejudice that arise in it constantly, here we may drink water and consume fruit.*

Who should practice this fasting of the mind? The answer is brief and simple, everyone! The entire purpose of the yoga practice is to silence the mind, to find some distance between our true self and our body/mind. The practice would involve that every time we catch useless thoughts arising within us, we let them go and remain mentally connected to Source and our guru through a mantra during this fasting period. When prejudice knocks at our door, focus on parapasata (deep breathing technique in which you hear a sound in you: mantra, guru mantra or seed mantra). Guru Baneshwaranand gives the following mantra to his students, feel free to make use of it as well. Ohm Brahma Swarupaya Baneshwaraya Gurubhyo Namah

3   *ASANAS (POSTURES)*

Postures in yoga are called Asanas, it is believed that a person should be able to sit in an asana for a minimum of 32 minutes. If he/she is able to accomplish this, it is called Asana Siddhi (achievement).

The meaning of yoga is union; union of what or to what?
UNION of self with higher self.

-And how does this happen? -
We achieve this by following the 8 limbs, in chronological order.

Asanas serve a specific purpose in supporting us in our alignment with the universe, making our body fit for the mastery of the higher limbs such as pranayama, meditation, and ultimately reaching the meditative state of yoga. At the beginning of the book we explain the lower limbs (such as non violence, etc.) The basic elements that need to be mastered before moving on to the higher limbs which we will cover in the following chapters. You cannot jump over a phase and think you will be successful. It is important to understand that in order to be well equipped to embody the upper limbs we first need to be well established within ourselves. We must first learn the restraints, and the observances before trying to take on the asanas and pranayama. This is how we can prepare ourselves for these higher realms without getting injured when these energies enter our body and rise to the crown chakra.

ASANAS (POSTURES)

How can we command our Prana or life? What is life? Ayama means exercising and Pran is life so it literally means exercising the life force.

There are over 70 Asanas, Shiva (the first yogi who ever existed) has gifted us with 10 main asanas. We should be able to master at least 1. Mastering is achieved by remaining in the respective position for more than 32 minutes.

Our human body is interconnected with our solar system, there is a great correlation between universal proportions and the structure of our bodies. Take the number 108 for instance. We have 108 chakras that need to be completely open for us to be able to receive and transmit effortlessly. Did you know that the distance between the sun and earth is 108 times the diameter of the sun, and the same applies to the diameter of the moon and the distance between the moon and the earth. We are made to align and resemble universal geometry. There are many more examples of how the solar system and the human body are intertwined.

Asana is a posture that was originally designed to be seated and still in general terms it is used for any seated meditation pose. Later reclining, standing, inverted positions and balancing poses were added as various types of yoga were developed.

We must always balance both legs and both hands during our practice because with that we balance feminine and masculine energies within, as Shiva represents the ultimate balance of masculine and feminine.

The asanas provide both spiritual and physical benefit and improve flexibility and strength in our body. Asanas will reduce stress and any adverse conditions related to stress. They are beneficial in treating some diseases like asthma and diabetes among many others.

Following are the 10 main asanas to practice and master, thereafter we will provide an additional 15 asanas in standing position, another 15 in sitting position, and 10 while lying on your belly and about 10 while lying on your back.

10 Main Asanas:

Swastikasana - Auspicious Pose

Swastikasana is a basic seated yoga asana often used in meditation, particularly when the yogi has difficulty with siddhasana and padmasana. The name comes from the Sanskrit, su, meaning "good"; asti, meaning "to be" or "existence"; ka, meaning "to make"; and asana, meaning "pose."

It's a beautiful meditation pose that stretches our lower body, it promotes spinal alignment and when the spine is stretched it strengthens our lower back. It provides all organs an optimal place to function and therefore when we meditate in this asana we get enhanced results in our practice both spiritual and physical. It also strengthens our root chakra, sacral chakra, third eye and crown chakra.

How to get into Swastikasana:

1. Bend one leg and place the foot against the inside of the opposite thigh.
2. Bend the other leg and place that foot in the space between the opposite thigh and calf muscle.
3. Grab the toes from the first leg and pull them into the space between the opposite thigh and calf muscle.
4. The spine should remain erect, and the hands should rest on the knees in a mudra such as jnana mudra or chin mudra.
5. Maintain a slow rhythm of breath.

Padmasana - Lotus Posture

The sanskrit word *padma* means lotus and *asana* posture, and therefore in English it is called lotus pose. It is basically a crossed legged posture which deepens our meditative state. We recommend the lotus posture for obtaining a deep meditation, and also as a means to alleviate physical ailments in the process. As we gain expertise in the lotus posture our life will also blossom like a lotus. The posture is an excellent workout for our body and mind as well as our breathing and with that it is considered the most important pose to master.

Padmasana increases our concentration and still calms down our brain resulting in enhanced focus and attention. It strengthens our root chakra and with that it solves various diseases and disorders related to the womb, regulates the menstrual cycle and improves the female reproductive system. It stretches our knees and ankles and prevents joint pain in elderly people, it assists with weight loss, it improves digestion, regulates blood pressure, and helps in childbirth.

How to get into Padmasana:

1. Sit down on the floor or mat with your spine erect
2. Bend your right knee and place right foot on left thigh
3. Bend your left knee and put it on top of right thigh,
4. Hold this posture and continue with a slow and long breath inward and outward
5. Stay seated for as long as you can

Gomukhasana - Cow Face Pose

Is it also called cow face posture, go means cow, mukh means face, and asana means posture. It provides flexibility to all joints: knees, thigh muscles, hips, shoulder joints, armpits, elbows and wrists. It stretches and tones the muscles of our chest, it enhances renal activity. It is also beneficial for diabetics and helps in sexual disorders and lower back issues like sciatica. It strengthens the nervous system and drives out stress and anxiety for optimal performance.

It's also available in some variations as vajra gomukhasana a higher level of yoga and maha vajra gomukhasana, baddha gomukhasana, hasta gomukhasana -they look like gomukhasana but are slightly more advanced. They are diamond cow face posture, great diamond cow face posture, bound cow face posture, and hand cow face posture respectively.

For optimal performance we are looking for it to look like a cow, your crossed legs should look like the mouth of a cow

How to get into Gomukhasana:

1. When prepping for this pose it would be useful to do diamond pose (vajrasana)
2. Sit with both legs out in front, bend the left leg and bring the foot under the right hip, bend the right leg put it on top of leg and draw towards the left hip in such a way that your right knee and left knee are on top of each-other
3. Without raising stay in a straight position and bend left hand behind and bring the palm up, raise the right hand straight bend down and reach to left as clasp hold it in this position
4. Close your eyes, breathe slowly and stay in this position for as long as you can

Virasana - Brave Pose

Also called brave posture or hero pose. Vira stands for brave, and asana for posture. The conventional meaning of hero is one who fights for the wellbeing of the world, he protects and safeguards the world from the enemy. In the context of our spiritual growth, the enemies are our inner demons such as fear, hatred, anger, frustration and ego, so the yogi hero is one who has overcome his own inner turmoil and makes others overcome their own inner turmoil.

It gives strength to our ankles, thighs and knees, improves and enhances the digestive health. It eases symptoms of menopause and relieves the swelling of the legs after or during pregnancy, enhances circulation of blood, and relieves us from leg pain, helps with stomach, high blood pressure and it helps with flat feet (specially for running).

All those with heart problems should avoid this posture. If you have any knee injury do not do it by yourself unless you are guided by a yogi.

How to get into Virasana:

1. *First kneel on the floor with your knees placed right under your hips,*
2. *Let your hands rest on your knees, then keep your knees together and open up your feet or widen them so much that they should become wider than the width of your hips.*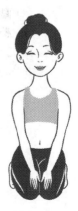
3. *Push your heels towards the floor*
4. *Lower your hips until they touch the mat on the ground, ensure that your hips are right in between your heels*
5. *Hold this position for at least 30 seconds or 5 breaths. There are 3 additional virasanas which are Supta, Dhyana and Laghu.*

Sinhasana - Lion posture

Sin means lion and asana means posture. It is beneficial when dealing with frustration, anger and stress to release negative energy from ourselves.

The benefit of this breathing technique is that it cleanses the throat and vocal cords, there is no other way to clean the mucus in your throat, it also alleviates bad breath. Please roar at least 3 times and keep your visual gaze on your third eye. Repeat as many times as you can.

Another benefit of this asana is that it relieves tension in your lungs, chest and face. There is a muscle called platysma (that connects mouth and throat) which is stimulated by this asana and consequently keeps the platysma firm through time. By practicing simhasana all 3 major locks which are called bandhas (mula, jalandhara, uddiyana) are engaged.

How to get into Sinhasana:

1. Kneel on the floor and sit in vajrasana, fold your knees and place your hands about 1 1/2 feet or 90 cm away from your knees- now your sitting position is like a lion
2. Take a deep inhalation, open your mouth wide and stick your tongue out, with eyes wide open, contract the muscles on the front of the throat and exhale with force making a distinct noise like haaaaa, the breath should pass through the back of the throat

Mayurasana - Peacock Posture

Muyur means peacock and asana refers to posture. It is an advanced hand balancing yoga pose, which strengthens our forearms, wrist and heart.

The physical benefits include detoxifying the body and ridding yourself of tumors and fevers, strengthening the digestive organs and increasing blood circulation in the abdominal area. This posture enhances our vision, dignity, prestige, sensuality, and generosity, It energizes the pancreas, stomach, spleen, kidneys, liver and intestines. Helps keep piles in check. It also strengthens and tones the reproductive system, reducing menstrual and menopausal dysfunction and improves sexual activity. Makes elbows, shoulders, wrist and spine stronger. Calms the mind, reduces stress and anxiety, helps concentration during mediation and improves motorized coordination between mind and body

How to get into Mayurasana:

1. *Sit on your heels with knees wide apart, place your hands on the floor*
2. *Let your fingers point towards your body, bend your elbows and press them towards the abdomen*
3. *Keep your belly firm, drop your head on the floor, and work up the strength in your stomach,* 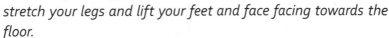 *stretch your legs and lift your feet and face facing towards the floor.*

Kukkutasana - Rooster Posture

Kukkut means rooster and asana means posture.

It enhances our mental power, therefore it enhances our ability to concentrate and focus. If we want to meditate we must always practice these asanas as it has all the properties of padmasana or lotus pose.

The benefits of this asana include broadening the chest, arms and shoulders building strength as well as focus, balance and stability. It enhances and activates muladhara chakra, stimulates the digestive system, reduces menstrual discomfort and pain. As it is an advanced posture we must beware of any conditions in the lung or heart area or any gastric ulcer, in those cases, always practice under supervision of a guru or teacher.

How to get into Kukkutasana:

1. *First sit in a padmasana, put your arms through your legs in the opening between the thighs and calf in such a way that hand touches the ground through this gap, push off your palm and lift your body.*
2. *As you lift your body, inhale, hold your breath and your body for as long as you can and then come down. You can remain in this position for 1 to 5 minutes or 1 to 5 breaths. Release pose with exhalation and return to the ground.*

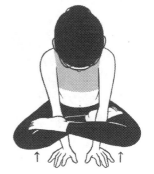

Bhadrasana - Butterfly or Gracious Pose

Bhadra stands for gracious and asana for pose, also known as butterfly pose. This is the best posture for meditation because it automatically takes you through your inner journey with ease.

It calms the mind, activates reproductive organs, activates the root chakra, strengthens ankles and knees, strengthens the spine, improves and supports the digestive system, helps with flexibility of legs, thigh, back bone, buttocks and hips. Regular practice will result in a healthy prostate and urinary system. It is beneficial during pregnancy. If you do this regularly labor will be effortless, helps ovaries and eliminates frigidity, helps in dissolving rectal diseases like hernia.

How to get into Bhadrasana:

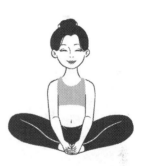

1. *We sit on the ground with knees bent and bring feet together*
2. *Supported with your hands, try to touch your knees to the ground, keep your head and neck straight, breathe gently, close your eyes.*
3. *Attention should be on your third eye chakra*
4. *Maintain this position for at least 5 breaths, then slowly stretch your legs again*

60 Kurmasana - Tortoise Pose

Kurma means turtle and asana meaning pose. Turtles are protected in all circumstances, so when we get threatened or alarmed we will always be protected with this asana.

Regular practice will result in improved flexibility of the body, it stretches the thighs and hips deeply and it also helps back, shoulders, chest and your upper body. We will feel total relaxation of body and mind.

How to get into Kurmasana:

1. *Start in seated position back straight with legs extended in front of you*
2. *Put your arms in front of you keeping them in between your legs*
3. *Lean forward, slide your arms out to the side with palms facing down, arms should slide under slightly raised knees*
4. *You stretch so much that your head and chin will start touching the ground, then extend your gaze ahead and allow your thoughts to shift from the external world to the internal world.*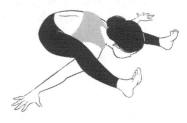
5. *Hold this pose for one breath then release the pose safely.*

Muktasana - Free Pose

Mukta meaning free and asana meaning pose. Frees us of all our worries. We sit as we want.

Improves flexibility, blood circulation, makes blood reach spine, stimulates your kidneys,

How to get into Pavan Muktasasana:

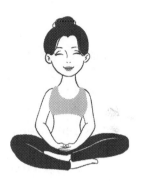

1. *Sit or lie down, bend your knees*
2. *Inhale slowly and fill all your organs with air*
3. *Hold your breath for some time and then slowly exhale completely.*
4. *Be as free as possible.*
5. *Repeat at least 3 times with 3 breaths each.*

Standing Postures

1 Tadasana- Palm Tree posture

Tada means Palm tree and asana means posture, even if it is commonly known as mountain pose in the west.

The body in this posture shall remain in the shape of a palm tree.
It is beneficial for energizing the nervous system, strengthening the heart and back bone, it activates your lungs, helps with weight reduction, and promotes growth in children.

How to get into Tadasana:

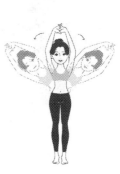

1. Stand straight with back bone erect
2. Stretch both hands above the head and open your palms in such a way that both thumbs join
3. Raise both heels and stand on your toes, stretching the whole body upward
4. Remain in this position as long as you can, breath slowly and normally
5. Release and relax

2 Vayuyanasana- Airplane posture

Vayuyan means airplane and asana meaning posture.

The body in this posture takes the shape of an airplane. Benefits include maintaining balance of body and mind, we develop concentration and body becomes buoyant.

How to get into Vayuyanasana:

1. *Stand up and stretch both arms along the side of the body*
2. *Bend forward from waist, raise your left leg backwards and straighten parallel to your upper body and perpendicular to your right leg making sure your knees are not bent.*
3. *Stay in this position maintaining the balance, breathing slowly and remaining comfortable*
4. *Come back to standing position and repeat with the opposite leg.*

3 Konasana - Angle posture

Kona means angle and asana means posture. It's a side stretching posture that stretches the sides of the body.

The body in this posture takes different angles. This asana reduces tiredness and stimulates the waist, legs and arm muscles.
Basically it stimulates the whole body.

How to get into Konasana

1. In standing position stand with both legs apart
2. Stretch both arms to the side making a 90 degree angle to the body
3. Inhale and as you exhale bend downwards towards one side raising one arm towards the sky and the other towards the floor.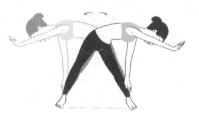
4. Breath in and come to the initial position
5. As you exhale, repeat towards the other side.

4 Trikonasana - Triangle Pose

Trikona means triangle and asana meaning pose. It's a foundation pose that is great for stretching.

The body takes the shape of a triangle in this pose.
Benefits include strengthening of the spine, waist, legs and thighs, helpful in weight loss and for all those with waist issues this is a great asana. Stimulates abdominal organs and relieves stress

How to get into Trikonasana

1. In standing position stand with both legs apart
2. Stretch both hands to the side making a 90 degree angle with the torso, 3.
3. Inhale and as we exhale bend to the side touching our right foot with our right hand while our left hand reaches towards the sky.
4. Inhale to center and exhaling as we reverse the side left hand to left foot
5. Repeat 10 times

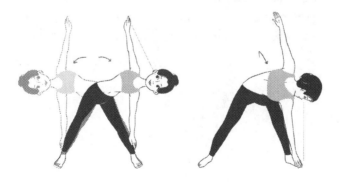

5 Uttanasana - Standing forward bend

Uttana means forward bend and asana meaning pose. It can be used as a resting position between all other standing poses.

It stretches every part of the body below the navel, it energizes leg nerves and strengthens the spine as the whole body weight pushes down on it.

How to get into Uttanasana

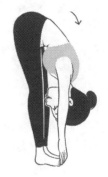

1. Stand straight, spine erect
2. Stretch both hands above the head and then exhale bending forward from hip joints (not from waist) therefore stretching the whole body.
3. Remain in this position as long as you can, breath slowly and normally.
4. Release and relax. Repeat 2 or 3 times

As you bend forward your focus should be on lengthening the front torso as you move fully onto the position, try to touch the ankles. Inhale and revert to initial position, exhale and bend forward for at least 3 breaths.

6 Vrikshasana - Tree Posture

Vriksha means tree and asana means pose. Great posture to enhance focus.

It strengthens legs, and balances your body, enhances concentration of mind, helps you become steady and grounded.

How to get into Vrikshasana

1. *Stand upright with both feet together touching the inner ankles and inner knees*
2. *Place the right foot on the left thigh, bring hands into prayer mudra and raise them up above your head, then open arms to the sides and back to anjali mudra (prayer position) in front of the chest*
3. *Repeat with opposite leg while breathing slowly*

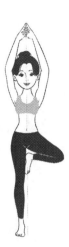

7 Surya Namaskar Asana- Sun Salutation

Surya meaning sun and namaskar used as salutation. It is the equivalent to namaste even if in normal tradition namaste was used for women to address their seniors and namaskar is really the term used among contemporary or people of equal age.

This Asana is all encompassing in its benefits, it takes care of all the joints in our body, as it is a combination of 12 yoga positions. It unwinds the mind and the body. It eliminates stress, boasts immunity, enhances the condition of the heart, is very effective for weight loss, improves digestion, and kidney function. It's practice results in beautiful skin among other benefits.

How to do Sun Salutation

1. Stand up straight, take your hands upward above the head and then exhaling bend forward and touch palms to the ground.
2. Inhaling take your right leg back, exhaling take left leg back to get into downward dog pose trying to keep both heels touching the ground
3. Inhale bend both knees to go into baby pose, exhale and extend arms in front as you lay forehead to the ground
4. Inhaling back up to go into cobra pose
5. Exhale and with both feet parallel to the ground
6. Inhale right leg forward, exhale bring other leg forward
7. Inhale go into tadasana, exhale and put your hands down to standing position.

8 Virbhadrasana - Warrior 1 Pose:

Virbhadra was the name of one of Shiva's servants who appeared in front of Shiva for the first time in this posture. This is how this posture got its name as asana means posture. It's one of the most powerful poses in the yoga routine.

The benefits include stretching of lower back, arms, legs, shoulders, neck, ankles, belly, groins. Energizes the entire body, opens the lungs, chest and hip, improves focus, stability and balance.

How to get into Virbhadrasana

1. *Begin by standing in upright position, step your right foot forward about 4 feet, keeping foot parallel and toes pointing to the top of the mat, bend your knee into a lunge.*
2. *Keep your left leg straight behind you and turn your left toes to a 45 degree angle*
3. *Raise your arms straight above your head and keep your shoulders pressed down.*

   The difficult part of this pose is to hold the entire body including shoulders, back, buttox and the left leg in a straight line

4. *Keep arms above the head, hands should always stay together*

Virbhadrasana: Warrior 2

We shift from one to the other by opening the arms. Here hands are to the sides of the body as opposed to above the head, rest of the posture remains the same

This pose stretches almost the entire body, you are able to balance the entire body on one foot.

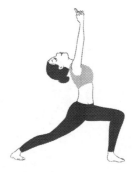

9 Ardha Chandrasana - Half Moon Pose

Ardha means half and chandra is moon, and asana is posture. It is a standing balancing pose, quite challenging for most people but of great benefit to enhance our focus.

Strengthens thighs and ankles by making thigh bones strong, strengthens spine, buttox and abdominal wall, it improves digestion, and balances your body.

How to get into Ardha Chandrasana:

1. *Stand straight as you do in Tadasana, place your feet apart from each other lifting one leg at a 90 degree angle from the other leg.*
2. *Lift one arm perpendicular to your body while keeping the other hand touching the ground, head should be kept straight farthest from the body.*

10 Natarajasana - Dancer Pose:

Strengthens chest, ankles, hips and legs, improves digestive system and calms the mind by releasing stress. Improves concentration and helps in weight loss.

How to get into Natarajasana

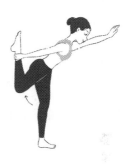

1. *Standing straight, arms by the side of the body, bend the left leg backward and hold the ankle with the opposite hand by moving the left leg upward as much as possible.*
2. *Extend the opposite arm straight in front of you, holding it for 30 seconds or 1 breath and slowly come back and repeat with the other leg.*

11 Hasta Padangushthasana - Extended hand to big toe pose:

A Major benefit is an increase in energy, and added strength in the legs.

How to get into Hasta Padangushthasana

1. *Stand erect, raise the right leg stretching it straight parallel to the ground*
2. *Hold the big toe of your right leg with the right hand and balance your body. Keep the position for one breath.*

*12 **Dhruvasana**- Tree posture with hands in anjali mudra*

Dhruvasana got its name from yogi names Dhruva who achieved enlightenment at the age of 5, during meditation he was able to chant and stay in this position for 6 months.

Benefits include improvement of concentration and reduced laziness, very good posture for meditation

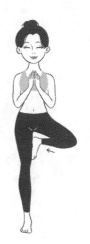

How to get into Dhruvasana

1. *Bend the right leg and place it on top of left thigh*
2. *Bring both hands to chest to anjali mudra, remain there for one breath and then repeat with the opposite leg.*

*13 **Vatyayanasana- Horse Face Pose***

Vaatayansana got this name from yogi Vaatayan who used to meditate in this position.

Benefits are multiple, it helps heal hernia, curves sexual appetite and prevents wet dreams, strengthens knees, waist and back bone.

How to get into Vatyayanasana

1. *Stand straight lifting the right foot and putting the right sole on left thigh*
2. *Then bend your left knee forward and place right knee close to the heel of the left*

14 Garudasana - Standing Garudasana

The benefits include the entire body, positive effects over the nervous system as it is stimulated and becomes active preventing ever getting any type of paralysis, relieves sciatica and hernia. It massages all organs as it's like twisting a rag and getting all water out.

How to get into Garudasana

1. *Stand up, crossing both legs and hands, keeping right leg on ground, lifting left leg up and turn around across right knee*
2. *Place left foot on right calf now bend right hand at elbow level and lift up, turn left hand across right elbow join hands in namaste mudra*
3. *breath slowly and repeat on the other side.*

15 Shirshasana - HeadStand pose

Benefits include regulation of circulation and nervous system, lung and heart function improves, sight is enhanced, memory is increased, diabetes and piles are cured.

How to get into Shirshasana

1. *Sit in a bhadrasana, interlock both palms, raise the entire weight of the body on hands and place hands on the ground raising the knees and slowly lift both legs upward*
2. *Stand on your head balancing for 1 breath, increasing up to 1 minute. Be sure to place a thick cloth beneath your head*

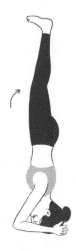

Sitting Postures

16 Padmasana - Lotus posture

Benefits include: It enhances awareness, strengthens our joints and reduces our anxiety, reduces menstrual discomfort, reduces insomnia, improves digestion and helps pregnancy and delivery

How to get into Padmasana

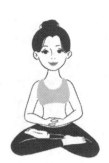

1. *Sit placing left foot to right thigh and left foot to right thigh keeping back bone straight*
2. *Close your eyes breathing as slowly as possible.*

17 Siddhasana- Accomplished pose

Also called meditation pose. Benefits include the same as Padmasana but not as strong as Padmasana.

How to get into Siddhasana

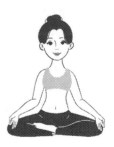

1. *Sit cross legged keeping both palms on your knees*
2. *Close your eyes and breathe as slowly as possible.*

18 Dandasana - Staff Pose

Dandu meaning stick and asana means posture, so sitting with a straight back like a stick is dandasana.

Benefits: Improves awareness, opens chest, leg and shoulders.

How to get into Dandasana

1. *Sit with straight legs, both feet touching in front of you*
2. *Place both hands on the side of the body touching your hips. Lift your body slightly with your hands in such a way that the weight of the upper body is resting on your palms, spine should be straight and stretched, breathe as slowly as possible. Keeping fingers in an open position.*
3. *Maintain position for 30 seconds at a minimum.*

19 Paschimottanasana- Seated forward bend

Benefits include strengthening of back muscles, calves, hamstrings.

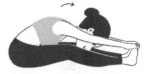

How to get into Paschimottanasana

1. *Sit with straight legs, both feet touching in front of you*
2. *Lift both hands up with open fingers, spine should be straight and extended, breathe as slowly as possible.*
3. *Maintain for 30 seconds at a minimum.*
4. *Lift arms towards the ceiling exhaling and bending forward over you legs till you touch your feet. Repeat 6 times, 6 breaths.*

20 Janu Sirsasana- Head to knee pose

Benefits include: stretches legs, inner thighs, hips and hamstrings.

How to get into Janu Sirsasana

1. *Sit with straight legs, both feet touching in front of you,*
2. *Lift both hands up with open fingers, backbone should be straight and stretched, breathe as slowly as possible. Maintain for 30 seconds at a minimum, bend your left knee and place the sole of your left foot on the upper right thigh, lift your arms and flex your right foot, exhale and bend forward to your right leg and hold your right toes. Take your forehead as low as possible breathing slowly and remain here for 2 or 3 breaths. Inhale and switch back to the other leg and repeat.*

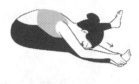

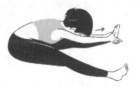

21 Vajrasana - Kneeling Pose or Diamond Pose

It is also called thunderbolt pose. It Improves digestion and regular practice eliminates constipation, reduces ulcer and acidity, helpful in sciatica and lower back problems. It strengthens our pelvic muscles, reduces liver pain and is very helpful in attaining meditative state.

How to get into Vajrasana

1. *First you kneel down, and sit on your calves so that the buttox is resting on your heels, calves and thigh muscles, keeping them together.*
2. *Place hands on knees and gaze forward, keeping your head absolutely straight and breathing slowly. Observe your breath as you inhale and exhale.*
3. *Close your eyes and concentrate solely on breathing, remain here for 3 breaths.*

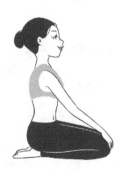

22 Sukhasana -Easy Pose

Even if it's easy it has amazing benefits, it opens the hips, eliminates fatigue, enhances comfort level and brings spine to a natural curve.

How to get into Sukhasana

1. *Sit in a cross- legged position*
2. *Tuck each foot under the opposite leg*

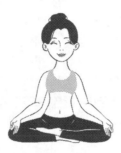

23 Baddhakonasana - Butterfly pose or Bound Angle Pose:

Benefits include stretching of inner thighs and opens up the hips.

How to get into Baddhakonasana

1. *Sit down and spread your knees bringing the soles of feet together and try to press the knees down to the floor.*
2. *Inhale and lengthen spine as much as you can and while exhaling imagine bringing navel towards your feet.*
3. *Repeat several times.*

24 Ardha Matsyendrasana - Half Spinal Twist:

Benefits include stretching your upper back, side body, pelvic muscles and spine

How to get into Ardha Matsyendrasana

1. *Sit in a cross- legged position, scoot your left knee towards the middle and place the sole of your right foot flat on the floor on the outside of your left thigh, right knee would be pointing at the ceiling.*
2. *Inhale and lift both arms overhead, exhale while twisting to the right placing your right hand on the floor behind you and your left elbow touching the right side of your knee.*
3. *Bring your left hand through your fingertips and press your right foot strongly on to the floor from heel to the tips of your toes. Now inhale and lengthen your spine, exhale and deepen your twist. Repeat for 5 to 10 breaths.*

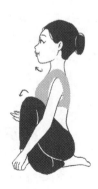

25 Nispand Bhavasana - Relaxation Posture:

Benefits include an enhanced feeling of peace and serenity, relaxes body and mind completely.

How to get into Nispand Bhavasana

1. Sit down and spread your legs 10 to 18 inches apart.
2. While leaving them relaxed place both hands behind your back, keep your head raised and breathe as slowly as possible as you mentally scan each part of your body

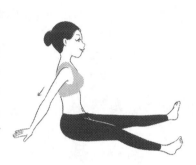

26 Padungasthasana- Sitting on your Toe Pose

Main benefit is the stretching of your toes, and provides all benefits such as stretching of thighs, ankles and calves. It enhances our concentration.

How to get into

1. Sit down, fold your knees and put weight on the body on knees and toes.
2. Breathe slowly and stay in this position for as long as possible.

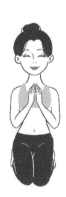

27 Ardha Padmasana - Half Lotus

Benefits of this pose include opening of the hips, stretching of the ankles and also the feet. Lotus is one of yoga's most important poses but not accessible to everyone therefore half lotus is there to transition you to full lotus.

How to get into Ardha Padmasana

1. *Sit in a cross-legged position, with back upright*
2. *Take the toe of one of your feet and place it on the opposite thigh, remain there for as long as you can. If you start feeling pain in your knee undo pose, otherwise stay here for 5 to 10 breaths.*

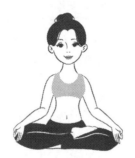

28 Balasana - Child's Pose

Benefits for this pose include stretching of the hips in a gentle manner, stretches thighs and ankles as well. Calms the stress and relieves fatigue, relieves back and neck pain. Great asana if you want to practice with your partner.

How to get into Balasana

1. *Sit in Bhadrasana touching your toes together and sitting on your heels, separate your knees as much as you can*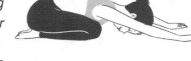
2. *Inhale and then exhaling lean forward taking your torso between your thighs.*
3. *Exhale coming back up and repeat 2-5 times.*

29 Malasana - Garland Pose

Benefits include stretching of the back bone, thighs, heels, ankles, and a calming effect on your nervous system.

How to get into Malasana

1. *Squat down with your toes and heels completely touching the ground*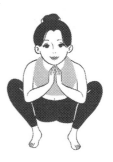
2. *Separate your thighs slightly at least wider than your torso and fit your torso between your thighs, place palms in anjali mudra, stay in this position for at least 2 breaths*
3. *Lean torso forward while exhaling till forehead touches the ground. Stay like this for 1 minute.*

30 Virasana - Hero Pose

Benefits include stretching of thighs, knees and ankles, improves digestion, releases gas from the abdominal area, beneficial during pregnancy as it reduces swelling of legs, controls blood pressure and asthma.

How to get into Virasana

1. *Repeat everything as in Vajrasana, then open your feet and lower the buttox to touch the mat or ground.*
2. *Stay here for 2 breaths.*

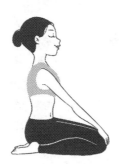

Lying Down Poses on your belly:

31 Bhujangasana- Cobra Pose

It enhances your memory. It is a miracle worker for the neck and waist, strengthens spine, lungs, heart and chest. Cleanses the uterus and regulates the menstrual cycle, reduces and avoids night semen discharge in men.

How to get into Bhujangasana

1. Lie on your belly, stretch your upper body while joining toes of both feet together, bringing both palms on the sides of chest
2. Inhale while raising the upper body such that the head is raised and looking up, exhale and come down
3. Repeat 3-5 times. If you find it difficult to achieve you can always use your hands to support yourself.

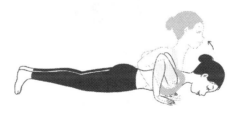

32 Shalabhasana - Locust Pose

Both large and small intestines get cleansed and therefore you avoid constipation, sciatica pain is significantly reduced, and pancreas function is improved. Strengthens lower abdomen.

How to get into Shalabhasana

1. Lie on your belly placing both hands under the thighs
2. Inhale and raise both legs, hold your breath and legs for 1 breath
3. Exhale slowly and bring down your legs. Your chin should remain touching the ground for the duration of the exercise. Do not bend your knees. For those who cannot lift both legs at the same time you can do 1 leg at a time.

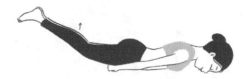

33 Dhanurasana - Bow Pose

This pose will get you all benefits you get from cobra pose and locust pose. This asana is very beneficial for women as it improves the reproductive system and urinary tract. Strengthens the spine, and reduces excess fat.

How to get into Dhanurasana

1. Lie on your belly, stretch your legs, bend legs towards buttox
2. Grab hold of your ankles with both hands, inhale and lift head, chest, thighs, hips, knees, legs and hands bending the body like a bow.
3. Stay here for 1 breath, repeat 3-5 times.

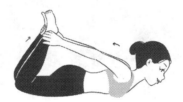

34 Vipareeta Merudandasana - Spinal Twist

Cleanses out your spinal cord of any energy blockages, improves lower back issues, reduces excess fat in the abdominal area.

How to get into Vipareeta Merudandasana

1. *Lie on your belly and stretch both hands to namaste position above the head or you can support your forehead with your hands*
2. *Joining both heels together and fold legs upward then sway left to right and right to left*
3. *Inhale and you go to center and exhale as you move from center to right and you move from center to left. Repeat 3-5 times.*

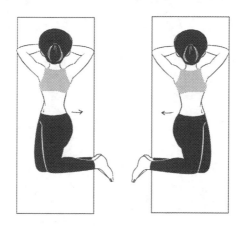

35 Nabhi Asana - Naval Pose

Our entire body rests on our naval hence the name. It strengthens the naval area as well as the entire abdominal region, keeps the naval in its proper place and empowers legs, hands and chest.

How to get into Nabhi Asana

1. Lie on your belly, stretch your hands and your legs, joining palms as in namaste mudra
2. Stretching both legs joining the heels. Inhale and raise hands, legs, head and chest to maximum possible height in such a way that entire body weight lays on your naval or belly.
3. Hold your breath and hold the position, and then exhale and return to the initial pose. Repeat 3-5 times.

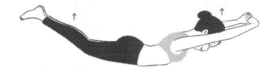

36 Kumbhakasana - Plank Pose

The main benefit is toning of muscles in biceps, thighs, abdominal area, reduces fatty tissue in that area.

How to get into Kumbhakasana

1. *Lie on your belly, lift your body such that only your toes and palms are touching the ground*
2. *Balance on your toes, face forward and down.*
3. *Hold for as long as you want. Repeat 3-5 times.*

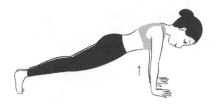

37 Makarasana - Crocodile Pose

Best asana to perform in the morning after getting out of bed and before you have dinner, and very useful for people operating computers, as it prevents back and neck problems and helps in spondylitis.

How to get into

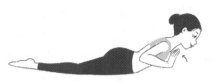

1. Lie on your belly, raise head and chest, take both palms and hold chin while elbows lay flat on floor.
2. Press your jaw and cheeks gently, breathe normally, close your eyes, and stay here for 2-3 minutes.
3. Release palm, lower head and relax. Repeat 2-3 times.

38 Shithilasana - Loose Posture

Rests the entire body, reduces tiredness, reduces tension, magical asana for those suffering from blood pressure and heart disease.

How to get into Shithilasana

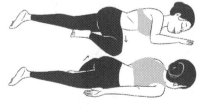

1. Lie on your belly, place your hands comfortably on the ground near your face
2. Turn your head to the right, bend your right leg, while keeping your left leg straight
3. Loosen your body, close your eyes and breath as slowly as possible. After 1 -2 minutes turn your head to the left, bend the left leg while keeping your right leg straight. Stay there for a minute.

39 Ardha Dhanurasana - Half Bow Pose

It strengthens the spine, chest and neck, and you get all the benefits of Naval, Cobra, Bow, and Locust Pose

How to get into Ardha Dhanurasana

1. *Lie on your back, join legs and feet and stretch your hands forward, hold right leg up and hold right ankle with left hand.*
2. *Inhale, lift your legs, head, chest, and hands as high as possible. Release and repeat with the opposite leg.*

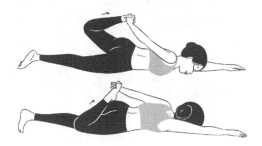

40 Vipareet Pavan Muktasana - Reverse Gastric Posture

Improves constipation, gas issues, acidity, stomach feels light and improves digestion.

How to get into Vipareet Pavan Muktasana

1. *Lie on your belly, place both hands under the shoulders on the ground firmly.*
2. *Inhale raising head and chest, fold right leg below the chest, exhale and touch chin to right knee, then inhale raising head and stretch right leg to normal position.*
3. *Repeat with the opposite leg. Repeat alternating both legs.*

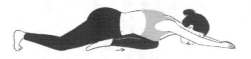

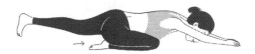

Lying on your back

41 Naukasana - Sailing Boat Posture

Strengthens sides of abdomen reducing fat, tones front tummy muscles, and strengthens the core.

How to get into Naukasana

1. Lie down on your back, feet together, arms on the sides, relax your shoulders
2. Slowly lift arms, chest and legs together off the ground. Reach 45degree angle so your body takes the shape of V.
3. Hold for 1 breath and lower and repeat 3-5 times.

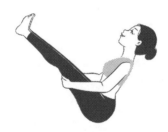

42 Sarvangasana - Complete body posture

As the name suggests this pose takes care of the whole body, it can be practiced by people of all ages. It strengthens heart lungs and brain, purifies blood, solves any issues in eyes, ears and mouth. Unwanted fat dissolves, digestion is enhanced. Neck and brain get energized, memory is enhanced.

How to get into Sarvangasana

1. Lay on your back, fold your knees in such a way that heels touch your hips
2. Lift and bend both knees towards the belly, give a little jerk holding your waist with both hands lifting your hips, shoulders, head and neck remaining on the ground.
3. Straighten both legs up and stay here for as long as you can.
4. Breathe normally keeping eyes closed, and after 2 min come to a lying position.

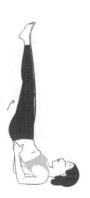

43 Urdhva Padmasana - Upper Lotus

Benefits are the same as Sarvangasana and Padmasana. Furthermore peace and calmness get restored. An indecisive and scattered mind gets settled.

How to get into Urdhva Padmasana

1. Lay on your back, fold your knees into lotus pose, lift the hip and give a little jerk holding your waist with both hands lifting your hips, shoulders, head and neck remaining on the ground.
2. Keep legs in lotus as you stay here for as long as you can. Breathe normally keeping eyes closed, and after 2 minutes come to a lying position.

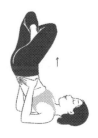

44 Halasana - Plough Pose

Benefits are multifold as it heals thyroid issues, heals diabetes, and hernias. It activates the uterus and is very useful for women who want to become pregnant, strengthens spine, hips and waist.

How to get into Halasana

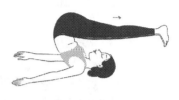

1. From your position of Sarvangasana you fold the body at waist level such that legs and feet lower until toes touch the ground, then your hands should be straight parallel to the torso.
2. Remain in this position breathing normally for 2-3 breaths, then come back to sarvangasana and then to normal lying pose

45 Karna Peedasana - Knee to Ear posture

Gives all benefits of Sarvangasana, and Halasana and in addition cures deafness and ringing of the ears.

How to get into Karna Peedasana

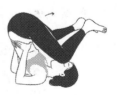

1. Starting from Halasana fold the knees until they touch ears and press ears a little bit
2. Breathe slowly and stay here for 2-3 breaths
3. Then unfold to Halasana, then to Sarvangasana and then to normal lying pose.

46 Chakrasana - Wheel Pose

Benefits include energizing the spine, lungs, stomach, hands and legs. Uterus problems get solved. Your brain gets enhanced as there is better blood circulation, it eliminates migraines, this posture also keeps you looking youthful.

How to get into Chakrasana

1. *Lie on your back, bend both knees, and bring your feet near buttox.*
2. *Bend your elbows placing both palms near your ears.*
3. *Touching your shoulders. Firmly press feet and palms towards the floor, inhale lifting the entire body upward*
4. *Stay here for a breath or 2 and come back. Repeat 3-5 times.*

47 Uttan-Padasana - Raised Leg Posture

It reduces gas, enhances appetite, cures back pain, enhances efficiency of heart and keeps the naval in proper place.

How to get into Uttan-Padmasana

1. *Lie on your back, stretch legs straight, place hands at side of the body with palms touching the floor, neck and head also rest on the floor*
2. *Inhale and lift legs to a 75 degree angle from ground, inhaling as you raise and exhale as you bring them down. Repeat 5-7 times.*

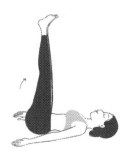

48 Balasana - Child's pose on your back

Benefits include strengthening of all joints in legs, knees, ankles, thighs and calves, and of course blood circulation is regulated

How to get into Balasana

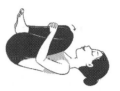

1. *Lie on your back, move legs and arms in the motion of a bicycle together with your head moving left to right.*
2. *Breath normally and after doing this for 2 minutes, reverse the action to backward motion for another 2 minutes.*

49 Hasyasana - Laughing Pose

Every benefit provided by Balasana also removes all stress from your body and mind.

How to get into Hasyasana

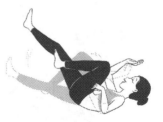

1. *While lying in childs pose on your back and moving arms and legs as described in balasana*
2. *Laugh hahahaha, hehehehe, hihihihi, hohoho, and huhuhuhu. The key is utilising every vowel.*

50 Pavan Muktasana - Gastric Pose

It flushes all impure gases out of the system, and solves all constipation issues. Regular practice reduces obesity. Spine gets strengthened and lungs function properly and knee pain gets relieved.

How to get into Pavan Muktasana

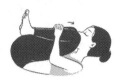

1. Lie on your back with legs straight, bend both knees and bring them to the chest holding them with your arms and exhaling as you hug them.
2. When exhalation is 100% complete, lift your head to your knees and kiss them. For those who cannot do both, try with 1 leg at a time in the same process.

51 Savasana - Peace Posture

Relaxing the entire body and eliminating mental fatigue, the body gets completely re-energized during this asana, therefore you will get up full of energy from it.

How to get into Savasana

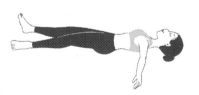

1. Lie on your back with palms looking upward, spreading legs slightly apart and loosening the entire body.
2. Breathe slowly and remain thoughtless, be very aware of your breath.

4

PRANAYAMA (BREATHING TECHNIQUES)

What is pranayama?

In simple terms, it is the magic of conscious breathing. The only difference between humans and animals lies in our consciousness. Even if we share the same basic activities like eating, reproducing, sleeping and breathing, we are the only species gifted with the power to exercise these activities in a conscious way.

*Conceptually, Prana is life and Ayama is to exercise, so in short, the ability to exercise life is called Pranayama. But what does it mean to exercise life? What a vague and ample concept you might think. Well actually it's so empowering and all encompassing. It's our capacity to balance, calibrate, cleanse and bring ourselves back into complete harmony when we stray away. We tend to gather daily energy through so many channels: through the air we breathe, the water we drink, the food we eat, the thoughts and emotions we allow ourselves to feel, and not all of the energy gets consumed completely. More frequently than not there is waste energy accumulated in our system that our body has not been able to make use of or discard. These accumulations of energies stay with us if we do not know the right way to release them. Each breath rids the body of waste, replenishes the bloodstream with oxygen, and thus nurtures our cells. The same way we release waste from food when we go to the bathroom, we must release waste energies stored in our **vayus, nadis and chakras through Pranayama.***

We tend to think that inhaling and exhaling is all there is to it, but that is an incomplete picture of the vast energy system that powers and fuels our body. In this system there are different mechanisms that make use of this Prana energy so that we, without having to employ conscious effort we are able to maintain all vital functions like digestion, sustain our body temperature, and cellular regeneration. This vital source of energy that is behind all life is what we refer to as the breath that keeps us alive.

Yoga divides this complex energy system into five subdivisions which are called Prana-vayus. Prana gives life and any disturbance in the Prana could cause the system to malfunction.

What are VAYUS?

Let's keep it simple, Vayu means air, breath, life force. There are 10 vayus present throughout our body, they are involved in all physical functions that pertain to the element of air such as breathing, urinating, defecating, hiccups, blinking, vision, digestion, exhalation, joint movement, hunger and thirst, opening and closing of heart valves, decomposition of the body after death, yawning, etc. Different types of air are responsible for different types of activities in the body.

The first 5 are called Pancha Prana which are most significant to the physiological human function and very important for the practitioner of Pranayama:

Prana Vayu absorbs vitality from the universe, and affects our vitality. Our main source of Prana clearly comes through inhalation, breathing air from the atmosphere and filling our lungs, we receive Prana as well through other sources such as water, food, sounds, sights, any impression that comes in through the senses. Prana is housed in our Heart and Third Eye Chakra.

Samana Vayu is mainly present in the digestive organs and circulatory system, it supports the fire element involved in digestion and it is usually present in the abdominal region. It is commonly associated with the Manipura or Naval Chakra,

Vyana Vayu integrates the prana vayu and all other vayus, nourishing our system. It governs the movement of prana through all 72,000 nadis (energy channels) that flow through the body. It is the force that distributes prana causing it to flow. Unlike samana, which draws energy to a focus at the navel center where it can be assimilated into the energy system, vyana moves energy outward to the peripheries of the body.

Udana vayu, "ud" which is the beginning of the word, connotes upward movement, such as the movement of energy in the windpipe for vomiting. It's responsible for our speech and communication as well as leg and arm movement and maintains our skeleton, muscles and joints as it is responsible for any upward movement like running and jogging. It has everything to do with the earth as it is responsible for the skeleton and it is made from the earth elements such as calcium. It is associated with Throat Chakra.

Apana vayu is related to exhalation and downward and outward movement. The carbon dioxide you exhale is called Apana vayu, and also supports all water functions and elimination functions like urination, reproductive functions like delivering a baby, defecation, etc. Apana has its home in the intestines and is focused at the Muladhara or Root Chakra.

Other relevant Vayus:

Kurma vayu, which is responsible for blinking and the opening of our eyes
Naga vayu is responsible for hiccups and burping
Krikala vayu is responsible for sneezing, hunger and thirst
Devadatta vayu is responsible for yawning
Dhananjaya vayu is responsible for the opening and closing of our heart valves and the decomposition of body after death

What are NADIS:

NADIS are energy channels through which PRANA – divine energy, life force and consciousness travel. On a physical level the Nadis correspond to the nervous system, they are drain arteries made of flesh and fibers inside the human body in charge of supplying pure blood and oxygen to all our organs from the heart, but their influence extends beyond this to the most subtle and spiritual level of our existence. The word is derived from nad meaning vibration, flow or motion, so nadi means something that flows like water. They are the energetic irrigation system which keeps a human alive. There are more than 3 1/2 million nadis but 72,000 (36,000 on the left side connected with main nadi Ida and 36,000 on the right connected with main nadi Pingala) are the most prominent ones of which 14 are the main ones we will focus on.

When all the Nadis are functioning correctly we are vibrating in health and happiness. But most of humanity suffers from either physical ailments or emotional distress, the result of Nadis being in a suboptimal state in need of balancing.

<u>Understanding the Nadi System</u>

Three Nadis are of special importance - IDA, PINGALA and SUSHUNMA.

- IDA arises in the left side of the body and represents the female, the Moon principle and water element. Its counterpart is the sympathetic nervous system
- PINGALA begins on the right side of the body and symbolises the male, the Sun principle and fire element, its counterpart here is the parasympathetic nervous system
- SUSHUMANA runs to the brain through the central channel of the spinal cord and represents consciousness, its counterpart is the central nervous system

Only when the moon (IDA) and sun (PINGALA) systems are in harmony in our body, we have a fertile ground for further spiritual growth.

The beauty of all this Pranayama work is that we are able to harmonize and activate the Nadis by our conscious breathing. In Pranayama through alternate nostril breathing we have an influence over our system, by breathing through the left nostril we will activate the Ida Nadi cooling and refreshing the system, while by breathing through the right we activate the Pingala Nadi which warms and stimulates. Just as the moon and sun determine cold and heat we have this built in thermostat which is in constant calibration. We can make use of it consciously or it can just run on autopilot. Our internal wisdom will activate as needed. When we are feeling cold we will start breathing through our right nostril to warm ourselves and when we are feeling hot we will breathe through our left nostril which has the opposite cooling effect. These Ida, Pingala and Sushumana Nadis are most prominent as they are responsible for the breathing process.

To maintain balance both of the side-Nadis (Ida and Pingala) run in a snake-like pattern from one side of the body to the other, overlapping the central line of Sushumana at 7 key points where they meet and where they generate powerful energy centers called Chakras.

The first chakra or crossing of the Nadis is at the base of the spine called the Root or Muladhara Chakra, and the last crossing point ends at the Pituitary /Pineal Gland called Third Eye Chakra. Each chakra is connected to all other chakras but more so to the previous and following chakra. We must create an environment that allows unobstructed movement of energy from head to toe, as only when this flow of energy is optimal we function at our full potential.

For the flow of energy to be optimal all 3 main Nadis should be active and flowing, so activating the Sushumna Nadi is of key importance. The Sushumna Nadi is compared to a sacred hidden river in India that only surfaces during certain planetary constellations, in the same manner this Nadi lies dormant in us most of the time and only awakens at dawn and dusk or during intense meditation. When the three main Nadis are flowing as one, the internal chatter or monkey mind finds rest, all worries and emotions dissolve and we are enveloped in the bliss of divine consciousness. Ida and Pingala represent the duality present in this world, the masculine and feminice aspects of life, logical and intuitive and it is only by bringing balance to these two that will make you effective in the world, and capable of handling life successfully.

Most people live and therefore die in one or the other. That is where the importance of Sushumna comes in. It is the central line representing space, the emptiness, absent of any qualities, which remains dormant until tapped by us consciously.

Sushumna is the most significant aspect of our human physiology and only when accessing this energy will life begin to work in accordance to our true nature. In subtle body terms, the sushumna nadi is the path to energize the seven chakras as it is the central channel that connects our root chakra with our crown chakra and the cosmos.

The Nadis and Chakras have 4 dimensions of energy: the physical, the mental, the emotional, and the spiritual. They are interrelated and overlap each other. These energies are the different dimensions of our life that need to be harmonized for all life to function the way it should be.

Chakras play an important role in balancing these energies, they keep our body and mind healthy, enhancing our immune system and our inherent capacity to heal ourselves.

And how does it happen? The chakras will be aligned, activated and clear as a result of our conscious breathing which purifies the system through the nadis. When we talk about purification we refer to the separation of negative elements from Raw-Pure energy. The idea is to filter the negative from what is Pure, so filtering the toxic thoughts, toxic food, negative words, destructive actions and emotions. And this is achieved through Pranayama! Incredible but true, The Power of Conscious Breath.

Now the real pranayama is one!
It consists of 3 parts Rechak, Purak, and Kumbhak.

Rechak is exhaling first before trying to refill yourself with new air, in order to start you should always empty yourself or what we call being "at zero", there should be no air inside your container before you take your first breath.

Purak is the first breath, after being "at zero", it's that first breath we take from the energy body and fill the stomach, lungs and legs down to our toes, you fill the whole body completely with air.

Kumbhaka is holding the breath inside as long as you can.

When you practice this sequence for some time with your eyes closed you will automatically experience the feeling of flying, the air will create a balloon effect making you feel light weight and at ease, slowly you can then release the air and start over. Most of the books available on the subject nowadays have the process completely reversed and opposite to the correct way it should be done, they start from Purak....

The reason being that you cannot fill a bucket that is already half full, the key is to empty the bucket before commencing the process!!!! This is the proper way to advance on your spiritual path and to achieve enlightenment.

The most advanced method of doing pranayama to achieve enlightenment is when we close all orifices of our body, then in this situation of kumbhaka the energy starts rising up and it goes through your Heart Chakra through the Sushumna Channel to your Crown Chakra and when it reaches the Crown Chakra you have attained enlightenment. The closing of these orifices is achieved through a method called locks (bandh) applied in different parts of the body mainly naval and throat.

The sound for rechak (first exhale) is Ahhhh, the sound for filling up with new breath is Uhh and the sound for kumbhak (hold it in) is MA, the joining of these 3 sounds makes Pranav, this is birth of ohmmmmm, the Pranav mantra.

This pranav Ohm is nothing but source, nothing but our higher self, nothing but some like to call God. Thus the proper way is to perform the practical pranayama by way of Rechak, Purak, and Kumbhak and no other way. When you start pranayama your point of departure should be void of air, you should inhale from the left nostril first (Ida) in for a 16 second count, hold your breath for 64 seconds before releasing in a 32 seconds slow exhale, then repeat with the opposite nostril.

The above mentioned time sequence follows the ratio of 1:4:2. You can choose any length of time, but 16 seconds is the minimum to be considered Pranayama level. When you are able to achieve it, you will feel light weight and as if floating above ground. Upon daily practice it is possible to experience your body actually lifting off the ground.

There are many types of Pranayamas, described in different religious books such as the vedas, but here we want to focus only on the 8 which are most significant.

If your aim is spiritual development only 1 pranayama is needed, as explained previously. We will now discuss 9 more pranayamas with tremendous physical benefits along with one explained earlier making it a total of 10.

1. ***Nadi Shodhan or Nadi Shuddhi (Alternate nostril breathing):*** It's similar to Pranayama. You start by sitting in a lotus or meditative posture, close your right nostril and breathe through your left nostril, then alternate. You do this by using your thumb on the right nostril, index on forehead and middle finger on left nostril. This is 1 round, you must do at least 3 rounds with no minimum of seconds. NO need to hold, just in and out. Air in from left out through right, then inhale from right and exhale from left. Benefits are among others that it cleanses nadis in the body, thus the name Nadi Shodhan, improves our circulation, therefore releasing stress, balances our body temperature, and enhances life span. Breathing is usually done through lungs and not through stomach

2. **Bhastrika (Fire breathing):** Start by sitting in lotus or meditative pose, back straight with shoulders relaxed. You can start with either nostril by closing one and breathing in and out as fast as possible and for as long as possible. Repeat with the other nostril. Benefits include the purification of our blood thereby releasing toxins from the body, regulates our nervous system and reduces fat, therefore enhances digestion, People who should avoid are those with hypertension, heart complication, hernia, and low stamina.

3. **Ujjayi pranayama (Victorious breath):** Inhale slowly through both nostrils, hold breath for as long as possible, exhale slowly with whispering sound, contracting air pressure, do it 2 or 3 times. Those suffering from heart problems should avoid. It stimulates thyroid, strengthens vocal cords, makes your lungs, chest and throat healthy and improves circulation.

4. **Surya Bhedana Pranayama (Sun penetration breath):** In every pranayama you should try to sit in a lotus pose. Left nostril represents the moon and the right nostril represents the sun. In this practice close your left nostril with index and middle finger of right hand then inhale from the right nostril, close the right nostril and exhale through the left, repeat this process always inhaling through the right exhaling from left and do it 10 - 50 times. The benefits are it warms our body by increasing energy level and shall be done when we are feeling cold or during winter. It improves and purifies our blood and improves digestion, it delays the aging process, all those suffering from acidity, hypertension and heart problems should avoid it.

5. **Chandrabhedan (Moon Penetration Breath):** Sit in lotus pose, keeping your back straight and shoulders relaxed. Left nostril is moon and right nostril is sun, therefore close your right nostril with thumb of right hand then inhale from the left nostril, close the left nostril and exhale through the right, repeat this process always inhaling through the left exhaling from right

and do it 10 - 50 times. The benefits are that it cools the body and heals heartburn, reduces temp during fever, ideally it should be done during summer, if you are suffering from low blood pressure you should avoid.

6. **Sheetali Pranayama (Refrigerant Breathing):** Sit in lotus pose or any comfortable pose like Siddhasana, Sukhasana or Vajrasana, keeping back straight and shoulders relaxed, close your eyes, breathe normally and relax the whole body then put the tongue on lower lip and roll the tongue in V shape form and inhale deeply through the mouth then close your mouth and exhale through your nose, you can start with 2 rounds and go up to 15 rounds. Benefits are it cools the body, cures acidity and reduces hypertension, solves any issues with indigestion, enhances your eyesight and health of eyes and skin. We should avoid it during winter and in cool temperatures.

7. **Sheetkari Pranayama (Cooling breath):** Sit in lotus pose, keeping your back straight and shoulders relaxed, hands on your knees, eyes closed. Join upper and lower teeth, then place front portion of tongue against front teeth, separate the lips and inhale from mouth making a chilling sound, retain breath for as long as possible and exhale through both nostrils, this is only pranayam that makes your teeth and gums healthy, and cools the body. Should be avoided if low blood pressure

8. **Bhramari Pranayama (Bee sound breathing):** Sit in lotus pose, keeping your back straight and shoulders relaxed, hands on your knees, eyes closed. Close both ears with index fingers of both hands, raise elbows to shoulder level, inhale deeply, retain breath for as long as possible, exhale deeply making a buzzing sound like a bee. Benefits are stress release and calming the body, makes voice pleasant and melodious, strengthens vocal cords, cures throat diseases and enhances concentration. For best results do upon waking up and before going to sleep. It can also be performed in another version in savasana pose

which is a resting pose, just by relaxing, taking deep breaths and making the bee sound as you exhale.

9. **Kapalbhati:** (Breath of fire) Sit or stand with a straight back, (preferably in lotus if sitting down), concentration is on exhalation. Fill your lungs and stomach with air and then exhale forcibly pulling your diaphragm up, inhale again and repeat. Repeat for as long as you do not feel pain in your back. 3 to 5 rounds. Benefits include weight loss, strengthens back bone, strengthens inner belly part, cleanses naval chakra, heals stomach and digestive issues.

MUDRAS:

In our pranayama practice we can incorporate Mudras to activate our life force and have a greater effect on the balancing of our internal energies.

Mudras help us link the brain to the body, they can soothe pain, stimulate endorphins, change our mood and increase vitality. They are hand gestures to activate our energy flow through our body therefore enhancing our yoga practice. Let's look into the function of the brain and how it relates to this topic. Our brain only understands through imagery, that is why when we are children everything is taught to us in the form of pictures and images; from numbers to fruit to animals, everything enters as a symbol that is to be registered as information in our system. The right hemisphere of our brain is rarely, not to say never, used 100%, it's the side of our brain that visualizes God, Source and/or our higher self. It cannot analyze, it only perceives symbols. Therefore, in our human attempt to conceptualize God we always try to create a picture in our mind by putting him either on a cross, we imagine him with a beard sitting on the clouds or in lotus pose as we try to create a visual we can relate to. Once it is registered within us it is difficult to go back from knowing what we know, that information is there to stay. All spiritual information works in the same way, once it is grasped and assimilated within us, it's there for life. Therefore...Enlightenment is for life.

All ancient prayers have some type of Mudra associated with them, for example the Namaste mudra, etc. Through this and other mudras we are able to make the connection to the right hemisphere in our brain, hence connect to our higher self and experience a broader perspective of ourselves and the universe. Our right brain is able to communicate in psycho-symbolic form with our higher self and give us a deeper insight than what we could understand intellectually. Our intellect clearly knows that 1+1=2, but your higher self sees the infinite potential in that combination 1+1=11 and what those numbers could even represent energetically at other levels of perception such as 1+1=1. One being our ultimate blending with Source, which is the meaning of the word yoga where we connect with our higher self, this is total union or oneness.

We have a precious and expansive subtle body extending beyond our physical body known as our energy body through which we experience energy flows via symbols. It is through this unseen veil that is part of us that we are able to enhance our journey within this human experience. This is why mudras play such a key element in our ordinary lives and serve us immensely when we are in the process of ascending on our spiritual path and want to elevate ourselves. As we have mentioned in the earlier chapter of nadis, we have 8.4 million energy storage points throughout our body and each time we practice a mudra we are applying pressure to one of these points, creating a reverberation of energy along that nadi.

What is a thumbs up? It's a happiness mudra. All hand gestures and symbols used by us serve the purpose to transmit and allow energy to flow through ourselves or to others. Very powerful messages and information are transmitted through these actions. When we are scared we cover our mouth, when we are in awe or love we bring our hands to our hearts, when we are surprised or in shock we grab our head or pull our hair out, when we are upset we give the middle finger. We don't realize all day long we are sending vibrational information to our system, to our cells, our organs and soul. Now ask yourself, what do you want to communicate - love or fear? Hatred or bliss? It's a constant choice we are making with our hands and body gesturing. Be wise, conscious and very aware.

We have the whole universe in the palm of our hands, LITERALLY! Every element in the universe is at the tips of our fingers. Everything is connected to our palms and feet, all points have a very direct connection to every part of your body.

Did you know that when we die, every line in your palm disappears, as our soul leaves that information leaves along with it and it is no longer imprinted on us.

Given this there is a science developed in India where through the printing and reading of the lines in our palms we can access information as far back and forward as 7 lives, as all realities are happening simultaneously. Any circumstance in life can be modified and corrected. Only 3 lines on our palms are permanent, all other lines can be enhanced and modified through consciousness and working on managing our life energies, empowering ourselves to direct our life.

We came here to experience life and to expand ourselves and the universe while we are at it, not to fix anything not to repent nor suffer misery. We are Source in its infinite perfection. We are everything and nothing as Source in everything and nothing.

This substance of nothing is present in every --thing, and nothing is ever so present in all nooks and krannies in our brain and body, in every living cell within us. Nothing can always be transformed into something therefore it is the most powerful element. What we call zero is our access to limitless possibilities.

Mudras have the capacity to change matter, they can have a very powerful effect on our body even when applied by another, that is where acupressure got originated. Obviously it's not as powerful and permanent as if it comes from within, as it is not activating your right brain. It is nonetheless important to know everything we do has an impact, on the same token consciousness is the real key. We need to be aware of the meaning of things and how and why we are making use of them. Spirituality is not about reading a novel or an instruction manual. Religion does not provide you with the key to the wisdom of life, rather experience and consciousness help us gain life wisdom. It has to be acquired organically and become part of your being.

What is the origin of mudras? How do we know about their meaning?

This wisdom is available to all of us in the universe in the form of resonating frequency. All souls that have passed through Earth and have been attuned to this frequency have accessed this wisdom called Vedas.

Intuition is nothing more than an energy match, depending on how much your energy has been enhanced you will have access to this wisdom and beyond. The objective therefore is to elevate our frequency to the highest level accessible to us at any given moment. Everyone of Einstein's discoveries or Mozart's music compositions, was nothing more than a frequency match. Every song that will ever exist already exists and every discovery that is ever to come about is all available in the universe waiting for someone to match up, resonate with it and download it like a computer.

So why are mudras important in our daily life you might ask? Let's begin explaining the difference between right and left brain, the right brain only learns by symbols and images that is why when we are little every word we are taught is shown in conjunction with a picture. Mudras are just that, symbols or geometric shapes that our subconscious mind understands intuitively. So for example as soon as the mind sees that you are doing dhyan mudra it will send a signal to our body to go into deep meditation. The use of mudras will enhance every aspect of our development as we will be able to focus better, quiet our mind and lead it in the direction our soul intends to go. These images stay imprinted in our subconscious and therefore play a permanent role in our life, being part of our hard drive here and forever more.

Without awareness mudras are nothing, and without mudras awareness is nothing. This connection mudra-awareness will enhance *your experience a million fold, making our yoga practice a blissful transcendental experience.* 🙏 *Namaste*

We have added some amazing Mudras here to enhance our life experience

Unmani Mudra

- *This mudra will mainly reduce anger, grief and calm our mind*
- *Helps us be centered in the present moment*

How to practice Unmani Mudra:

1. *Start in lotus pose, take a deep breath and hold your breath*
2. *Focus your awareness on a dot in the back of your head for as long as you can*
3. *While exhaling (kumback) keep your awareness on that dot which is on the back of your head, and then take your awareness to your spine from your crown chakra to root chakra.*
4. *Start at crown chakra with your eyes closed, and by the time you reach root chakra your eyes should be completely closed*
5. *Repeat process 5 times*

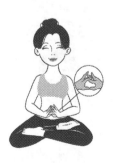

Shakti Chalini Mudra

–   Very helpful with all diseases related to the rectum such as hemorrhoids.
–   Helps in healing sexually transmitted diseases
–   Makes semen move upward therefore relieving impotence at the source of the problem
–   Stops aging process

How to practice Shakti Chalini

1. Start in padmasana or sidhasana with an erect spine, take a cloth of about 5 to 6 inches wide and wrap it around your waist. Put both palms on the ground 20 to 25 times, and then practice Mula Bandha and then Jalandhar Bandha
2. Kundalini is called shakti, it should start at the root chakra and the way to raise it to the crown is by pulling the energy with your breath and intention as you lock your root chakra or your sphincter in a rhythmic way. It involves contracting of the anal muscles.
3. It directs your prana upward along your spine and this prana energy is Shakti.
4. Practice 15-20 times and follow with a meditation of at least 5 minutes

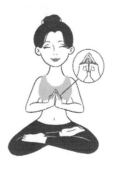

Kshepana Mudra

- *Drains negative chi from our body and attracts fresh new energy flow for optimal health*
- *Detoxifies us from stress*
- *Strengthens optimistic thoughts, releases frustration and irritation.*
- *Helps us to let go of all emotional heartbreaks and worries*

How to practice Kshepana Mudra

1. *Sit in Lotus*
2. *Clasp your hands as if in prayer, fold all fingers except index which should be straight and against each other, then place thumbs in the hollow area of the opposite hand*
3. *Ensure index fingers are pointing towards ground*
4. *This hand gesture should be downwards touching your body at sacral area level*
5. *Hold mudra for 5-7 breaths, focus should be on exhalation which should be slow controlled.*

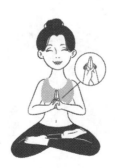

Mushti Mudra

- *Releases all irritation and calms anger*
- *Promotes a worry free state of being*
- *Activates digestion, reduces constipation, discharges unexpressed emotions*
- *Removes negative emotions*
- *Lowers high blood pressure, relieves heart complaints*

How to practice Mushti Mudra

1. *Sit in lotus, eyes closed, spine erect.*
2. *Place your hands in a fist on top of your knees facing down.*
3. *Press your fists on your knees and release for about 15 times*
4. *Breathe slowly*

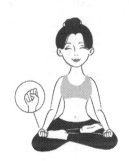

Gyan Mudra

- Strengthens our inner Wisdom and its capacity to expand
- Stimulates root chakra, reduces depression and tension
- Helps spiritual openness, enhances meditation
- Removes anger

How to practice Gyan Mudra

1. Sit in lotus, eyes closed, spine erect
2. Place hands on knees, joining tips of index and thumb while forming a circle and stretching remaining 3 fingers
3. Inhale and exhale deeply, stay here for at least 7-10 breaths
4. Your awareness should remain focused on your prana

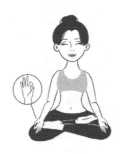

Pran Mudra

— *Provides effortless flow of prana (increase in prana reduces fatigue)*
— *Aids with insomnia, stimulates and enhances immune system*

How to practice Pran Mudra

1. *Sit in lotus, eyes closed, spine erect*
2. *Place your hands on your knees and then join the tips of the ring finger, little finger and thumb of each hand to form a circle. Stretch remaining 2 fingers*
3. *Inhale and exhale deeply, stay here for 7-10 breaths*
4. *Your awareness should remain on your breath*

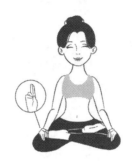

Buddhi Mudra

- *Enhances intuition, develops clear communication*
- *Relaxes your muscles and relieves muscular pain*
- *Useful for dry eyes and dry mouth as well as for kidney and bladder health*
- *Eliminates confusion, activates brain power and memory*

How to practice Buddhi Mudra

1. *Sit in lotus, eyes closed, spine erect*
2. *Place your hands on the knees and then join the tips of the little finger and thumb of each hand to form a circle. Stretch remaining 3 fingers*
3. *Inhale and exhale deeply, stay here for 7-10 breaths*
4. *Your awareness should remain on your breath*

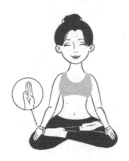

Rudra Mudra

- *Enhances body energy level, therefore earth element becomes stronger within*
- *Removes weakness, laziness and lethargy,*
- *Removes sadness, depression or any state of unhappiness*
- *Enhances spleen pancreas chakras*

How to practice Rudra Mudra

1. *Sit in lotus, eyes closed, spine erect*
2. *Place your hands on the thighs and then join the tips of the index, ring finger and thumb of each hand to form a circle. Stretch remaining 2 fingers*
3. *Inhale and exhale deeply, stay here for 7-10 breaths*
4. *Your awareness should remain on your breath*

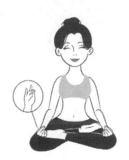

Surya Mudra

- *Provides benefit of sun energy, increases metabolism and digestion of food*
- *Enhances heat in your body, very useful in the winter season*
- *Enhances the fire element in your body, reduces body fat.*
- *Improves vision*

How to practice Surya Mudra

1. *Sit in lotus, eyes closed, spine erect*
2. *Place your hands on the knees and then press the knuckle of the ring finger down towards the palm of each hand. Stretch the remaining fingers*
3. *Inhale and exhale deeply, keep finger pressed for 7-10 breaths*
4. *Your awareness should remain on your breath*

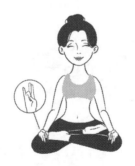

Apana Mudra

- *Regulates menstrual cycle*
- *Detoxifies the body*
- *Balances space and earth element within us*
- *improves digestion, very good for pregnant women for childbirth*

1. *Sit in lotus, eyes closed, spine erect*
2. *Place your hands on the knees and then touch tips of ring finger, middle finger and thumb to form a circle. Stretch the remaining fingers*
3. *Inhale and exhale deeply, stay here for 7-10 breaths*
4. *Your awareness should remain on your breath*

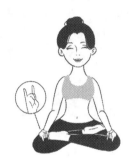

Shambhavi Mudra

- Enhances quality of meditation
- Helps us experience higher states of consciousness

How to practice Shambhavi Mudra

1. Sit in lotus and perform Gwhileyan Mudra
2. Focus your attention between your eyebrows or third eye
3. Stay here in this position for as long as you can, if your eyes start to hurt you should take a break
4. Your focus will automatically form an imaginary V shaped line having a dip in the eyebrows

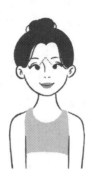

Vajroli Mudra

- *Eliminates problems of early ejaculation and unwanted night wet dreams*
- *Enhances immune system*
- *Semen moves upward to sacral chakra and person can be celibate or experience orgasm without ejaculation*
- *Intercourse lasts longer*

How to practice Vajroli Mudra (for men)

1. *Sit in padmasana or vajrasana, breathe normally with your spine erect*
2. *Pull up muscles around penis area, focusing your attention there. Pull upward towards the naval area for as long as you can hold and then release. When you pull your muscles up your breath will automatically stop for that period of time.*
3. *Exhale totally, perform abdominal lock, meaning pulling abdominal muscles inward and upward. Then add chin lock (jalandhara) to avoid any air coming in through nose and mouth. It helps to put your hands on the knees.*
4. *It feels like holding the urge to urinate*
5. *Repeat 15-20 times*
6. *Lie down on your back and perform boat posture (Naukasana), and repeat the whole process*
7. *Do it under expert or guided supervision*

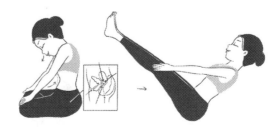

Sahjoli Mudra (for women)

- Promotes multiple orgasms and helps control compulsive sexual disorder
- Moves kundalini shakti upward towards crown chakra
- Tones uro-genital region regulating the functions.

How to practice Sahjoli Mudra

1. Sit in padmasana or vajrasana, breath normally with your spine erect
2. Pull up muscles around vagina area, focusing your attention there. Pull upward towards the naval area for as long as you can hold and then release. When you pull your muscles up your breath will automatically stop for that period of time.
3. Exhale totally, perform abdominal lock, meaning pulling abdominal muscles inward and upward. Then add chin lock (jalandhara) to avoid air coming in through nose and mouth. It helps to put hands on the knees.
4. It feels like holding the urge to urinate
5. Repeat 15-20 times
6. Lie down on your back and perform boat posture (naukasana), and repeat the whole process
7. Do it under expert guided supervision

Amaroli Mudra

– *Used for sealing vital energy within our physical and energy body*
– *Enhances Prana energy and moves kundalini upwards very fast towards our crown chakra*

How to practice Amaroli Mudra

1. *Sit in lotus, exhale completely and then practice uddiyan bandha to avoid air coming in.*
2. *Contract and release, contract and release your anal muscles 15-20 times as you pull belly inward and upward*

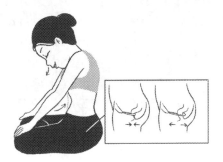

Vayu Mudra

- *Helps in weight loss and balances our air (prana, apana, vyana udana), reduces gas and pain related to flatulence*
- *Enhances happiness*
- *Relieves stiff neck and chest pain*
- *Builds immunity and protects us from respiratory issues*

How to practice Vayu Mudra

1. *Sit in lotus, eyes closed, spine erect*
2. *Start deep breathing, then press the knuckle of your index finger with your thumb towards your palm*
3. *Stay here for 7-10 breaths*

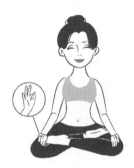

There are a wide variety of helpful mudras that can assist us in our life path. Anyone interested in going deeper can always contact the author of this book.

Balancing the Chakra System

Energy is everything and our capacity to perform anything physical or subtle is dependent on the quality of energy we are housing within ourselves. There are 8.4 million storage points in our system but 7 of these are the main ones to take into account and these are called chakras. They are present in us in subtle form, they are not physical. Every emotion present in us, positive or negative qualities are stored in the chakra system. Usually when they are open everything in our life physically, mental and emotionally flows effortlessly, in the same way when they are blocked we struggle in the various aspects of our day to day. Therefore when we are not feeling in optimum state we must look at this system, and seek to correct the un-balance present.

Our goal is to provide here all wisdom needed for us to recalibrate ourselves into alignment. I will explain the nature of each chakra, the emotions that govern and get stored within them, the mantras to heal, the stones to help balance, the sound vibrations and frequencies that resonate and therefore balance each chakra.

MULADHARA CHAKRA
The Root Chakra – the right to be here

Mantra: LANG power (fear)
Element: earth
Sense: smell
Planet: earth, saturn
Frequency: 360 Hz

Petals: 4

वं

VANG
vaṁ
joy (misery)

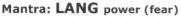

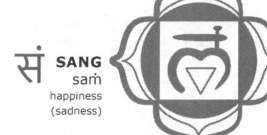

सं **SANG**
saṁ
happiness
(sadness)

SHANG शं
śaṁ
pleasure (pain)

KHANG
ṣaṁ
passion (insensitivity)

Asanas

षं

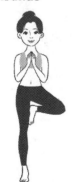

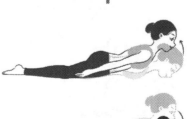

Gyana mudra

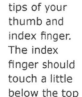

Connect the
tips of your
thumb and
index finger.
The index
finger should
touch a little
below the top
of your thumb.

Vrksasana
tree pose

Bhujangasana
cobra pose

SWADHISTHANA CHAKRA
The Sacral Chakra – the right to feel

Mantra: VANG   pleasure (guilt)
Element: water
Sense: taste
Planet: mercury, jupiter, moon
Frequency: 417 Hz

बं

Petals: 6

BANG
baṁ
sensuality (asceticism)

लं

LANG
laṁ
sexual phantasies
(actuality)

BHANG
bhaṁ
self-acceptance
(self-rejection)

भं

रं

RANG
raṁ
creativity
(destructivines)

MANG
maṁ
intimacy
(separation)

मं

YANG
yaṁ
sexual pleasure (guilt)

यं

Asanas

Pada Hastasana
hand to feet pose

Shalabhasana
locust pose

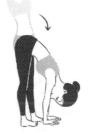

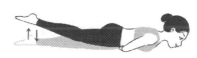

Dhyana Mudra

Rest your
hands in your
lap, palms fa-
cing up, right
hand on top of
the left hand.
Touch the tips
of your thumbs
gently together.

MANIPURA CHAKRA
The Navel Chakra – the right to act

Mantra: RANG   will power, (shame)   **Petals:** 10
Element: fire
Sense: sight
Planet: sun, mars
Frequency: 528 Hz

डं
DANG
ḍaṁ
cariosity (spiritual ignorance)
prana vayu

फं

दं

phaṁ **PHANG**
happiness (sadness)
dhananjaya vayu

DHANG dhaṁ
apathy (neediness)
apana vayu

पं

णं

paṁ **PANG**
cleverness (foolishness)
krikala vayu

NHANG ṇaṁ
acceptance (jealousy)
udana vayu

naṁ **NANG**
reality (illusion)
devadatta vayu

TANG taṁ
intimicy (treachery)
samana vayu

नं

तं

dhaṁ **DHANG**
phantasies (disgust)
kurma vayu

THANG thaṁ
pleasure (shame)
vyana vayu

DANG
daṁ
creativity (fear)
naga vayu

धं

दं

थं

Hakini Mudra

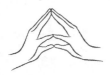

Put your hands before your stomach, slightly below your solar plexus. Straighten your fingers and put your fingertips together making a tent position, fingertips pointing away from your body. Cross your thumbs, left thumb over right thumb.

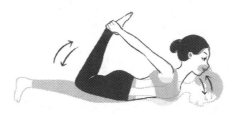

Asanas
Dhanurasana
bow pose

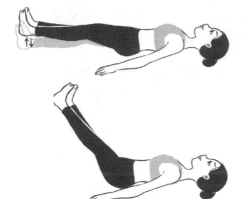

Uthanpadasana
raised legs pose

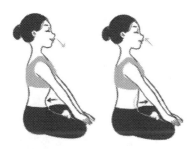

Pranayama
Kapalabhati

ANAHATA CHAKRA
The Heart Chakra – the right to love and be loved

Mantra: **YANG**   love (grief)   **Petals:** 12
Element: air
Sense: touch
Planet: venus, sun
Freqency: 639 Hz

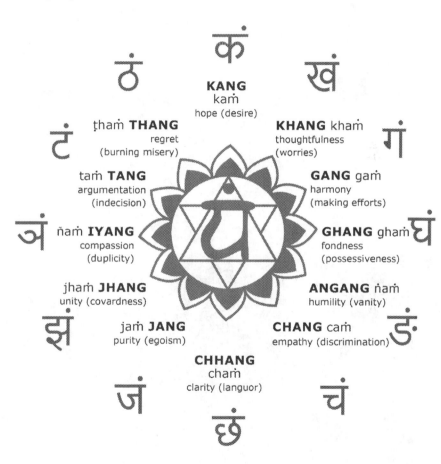

ठं   कं   खं

KANG
kaṁ
hope (desire)

KHANG khaṁ
thoughtfulness
(worries)

टं   ṭhaṁ **THANG**   गं
regret
(burning misery)

taṁ **TANG**   **GANG** gaṁ
argumentation   harmony
(indecision)   (making efforts)

ञं   ṅaṁ **IYANG**   **GHANG** ghaṁ   घं
compassion   fondness
(duplicity)   (possessiveness)

jhaṁ **JHANG**   **ANGANG** ṅaṁ
unity (covardness)   humility (vanity)

झं   jaṁ **JANG**   **CHANG** caṁ   डं
purity (egoism)   empathy (discrimination)

CHHANG
chaṁ
clarity (languor)

जं   छं   चं

117

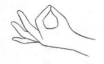

Gyana Mudra

Let the tips of your index finger and thumb touch. Put your left hand on your left knee and your right hand in front of the lower part of your breast bone (so a bit above the solar plexus).

Asanas

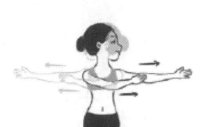

Trikonasana
triangle poses

Shukshma Ajam
hull rotation

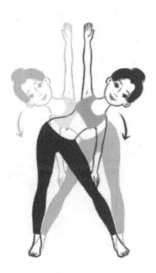

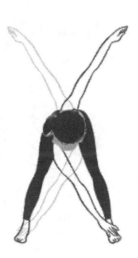

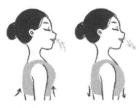

Pranayama
Bhastrika

VISHUDDHA CHAKRA
The Throat Chakra – the right to speak and hear truth

Mantra: HANG communication (untruthfulness) **Petals:** 16
Element: ether, space
Sense: touch, hearing
Planet: mercury
Freqency: 741 Hz

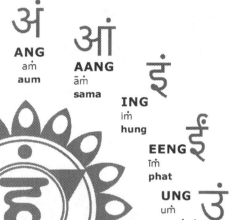

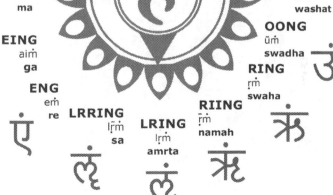

Emotions end in this chakra. The petals correspond to the vrittis of the mantra.

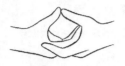

Vishuddha Mudra
Cross your fingers on the inside of your hands, without the thumbs. Let the thumbs touch at the tops, and pull them slightly up.

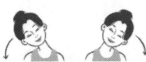

Asanas

Greeva Sanchalana
neck movements

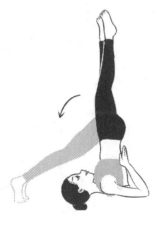

Sarvangasana
shoulder stand

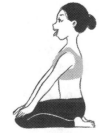

Pranayama
Swana Pranayama
dog breath

AJNA CHAKRA
The Third Eye Chakra – the right to see

Mantra: OM intuition (illusion)
Element: -
Sense: brain, neural
Planet: saturn, moon
Freqency: 852 Hz

✓ no more emotions
✓ only the power of mantra and music
✓ feminine and masculine consciousness united
✓ sound of the third petal appears when
  chakra is open

HANG
haṁ
(masculine)

KSHANG
kshaṁ
(feminine)

Kaleshwari Mudra
Put your hands before the lower part of
your breast. The middle fingers are straight
and touch at the tops, pointing forward.
The other fingers are bended and touch
at the upper two phalanges. The thumbs
point towards you and touch at the tops.

Asanas

Drishti Bheda (Alokita)
eye movements

Pranayama
Anulom Vilom
alternate nostril breathing

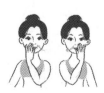

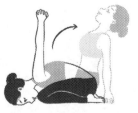

Vajrasana III
thunderbold pose variation

SAHASRARA CHAKRA

The Crown Chakra – the right to know

Mantra: No mantra - enlightenment (attachment)   **Petals:** 1000
No element, no sense
Planet: the whole universe, uranus
Freqency: 963 Hz

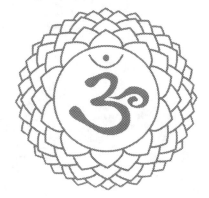

Chakra Mudra
Put your hands before the lower part of your breast. The middle fingers are straight and touch at the tops, pointing forward. The other fingers are ben-ded and touch at the up-per two phalanges. The thumbs point towards you and touch at the tops.

Asanas

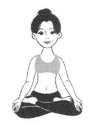

Pranayama
OM chanting

Padmasana/Sukhasana
lotus pose

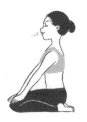 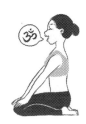

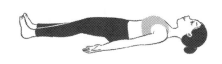

Savasana
corpse pose

5 PRATYAHARA (WITHDRAWAL OF THE SENSES)

We have completed the first 5 limbs of yoga which are considered the external aspects of the Yoga practice, better known in sanskrit as Bahiranga. From here on, we dive into the internal aspects of yoga called Antaranga.

Pratyahara is the first step into the inner phase of the yoga progression, ahara meaning food or anything we bring into our body and prati meaning away or against, therefore leaning away or withdrawing from any external distraction that stimulates the senses. When done appropriately it even has the potential to reduce hunger and quench our thirst.

The human body has 5 senses (taste, touch, sight, smell, and hearing). Our consciousness lies in that internal part of us where we no longer experience these senses. This non experiencing of our outer senses is called Pratyahara.

We must be able to bring all external experiences inward and experience them within us. Do you know that the mind does not know the difference between an outer event and an inward experience. If you laugh for no reason for more than 2 minutes you will produce the same hormones of happiness and joy as you would if you were laughing as a consequence of the funniest event ever. The same happens if we imagine a lemon with our eyes closed, our mouth will start generating the same digestive enzymes as if we were actually eating a lemon. The mind does *not have a mind of its own, it reacts to what we put in it, therefore we have complete control every minute of every day over our state of being.*

And how do we do this? We achieve it by controlling our senses, which can be achieved by mastering pranic energy. Pranic energy is what drives the senses, therefore if you want to stop the scattering of your vital energy you must start controlling its flow. It can be done through various practices by bringing the entire focus to one of the energized 18 points in our human body. These 18 points are distributed all over your body starting from both big toes all the way to the top of the head.

When we are in our pranayama breathing and we are in pratyahara, we start focusing on our toes, inhaling thinking that air is there on your toes, then moving this energy up your body through the root, naval, heart, and throat chakra and onward to the tip of the nose then center of eyes, center of eyelids, then forehead, until finally arriving at the crown chakra. The process is completely internal and should not take more than 30 minutes.

The first limbs of yoga are all centered on the physical plane, but once you have mastered the niyamas, asanas and pranayama through this systematic process of the first limbs the next phase which involves the inner journey will be easily accessible. Without this preparation as described above it would take 30 lifetimes to achieve. All ensuing practices up to the meditative state will take place internally.

When we are in Pratyahara, we are in a state of non reaction. The guidance of a spiritual teacher will be most helpful in this part as he will be able to influence us through the clarity of his intention. The best way it can be achieved is through savasana. There are a few things we don't see but can only experience, such as truth (reality) self (atma) brahma (source) and consciousness. They cannot be perceived through the senses. Our senses can only convey to us the outside world, so in order to experience our inner universe we need to disconnect from our senses or become unaffected by them.

How do we do this? How to withdraw from our senses?

*This aspect of withdrawal and controlling the senses is called **Indriya Pratyahara**. The best way to attain it is through savasana. Close your eyes very lightly or in such a way that your upper eyelid touches your lower eyelid only slightly. Relax your jaw, touch the roof of your mouth with tongue behind upper teeth, bring your attention to the root of your nose. With practice you will find it very relaxing, focusing here relaxes your sense of smell, relaxes your inner ears and you will begin to notice that your inner ears are tension free, and lastly relax your face, focus on your forehead and move your concentration on different parts of the face: eyelids, lips, neck, and then slowly slip into deep silence. There is no problem if you fall asleep, it is actually considered a very positive sign. It's a bridge between outer and inner journeys. It can be done laying down or sitting in lotus pose.*

*The control of senses requires mastery over the flow of prana because it's the pranic energy that drives the senses. In the absence of oxygen the senses seize to exist therefore we must harmonize the vital energy present in our body and not allow the scattering of it throughout, concentrating its entire focus on one chakra, one chakra at a time, this practice is known as **Prana Pratyahara**. It is with the power of our focus that we are able to direct the energy and concentrate it in a particular area of our body, it is the conscious control of life force. Do not try to visualize anything, focus on nothingness. Let's start with Prana Pratyahara which is pulling the prana air from different parts of our body and guiding it to reach the center of the 18 energized areas in our body: the first being the big toe of both feet, second is ankles, third middle of the thighs, forth is root of the tongue, fifth is knees, sixth is starting point of spine, seventh is root chakra, eighth is centre point of the spine, ninth is naval, tenth is heart chakra, eleventh is vocal cords, twelfth is root of palate, thirteenth is tip of the nose, fourteenth is root of the nose, fifteenth is center of the eyes, sixteenth is middle of the eyebrows, seventeenth is forehead and eighteenth is crown.*

*This practice not only involves control of the organs, but absence of actions including mental actions which is called **Karma Pratyahara** this leads to withdrawal of the mind consciously from anything to nothing* and that is considered the real Karma Yoga which is to surrender every action to our higher self and therefore allow the divine in us to be the one to perform every action, only as an act of service. Let's take a simple example like washing our family's clothes, we do it happily as it is Source experiencing this action through me, I do it for the mere pleasure of providing life or Source with the experience. Pratyahara is not about removing yourself from the world, it is something different as you see every action as inspired by a higher power. It means that even if I partake in the task at hand I am not vested in the outcome, upset by it or in displeasure. I will choose to enjoy everything I do as it is not me, it is the source of life doing it through me, that is the distinction. My actions are always being surrendered to the divine, I see every action as a divine action being performed by a higher power. Every mundane action is important, even washing the dishes I enjoy thoroughly as it is not me but the Source of creation experiencing this moment. As long as you have a body you cannot be action free, all you can be is in the state of allowing life to flow through you and witnessing the moment as perfection. Every moment should be a divine moment.

Withdrawing our senses, our Prana, our Karma inward is called Mind Pratyahara. And when we withdraw everything: senses, prana, karma and our mind that is the real Pratyahara.

Lastly we have Mano or Mind Pratyahara....what do you do with your mind? Our mind always wants to do something, that is because it's continually interested in achieving results. Even within the practice of Prana Pratyahara the mind is thinking it will increase it's levels of concentration, so there is always mind activity. When you are no longer involved in the results you will be able to achieve Mind Pratyahara. Only when you have successfully achieved Indriya, Prana, Karma only then will you be a container capable of experiencing Mano Pratyahara.

We can even achieve the results of physical rituals such as fire rituals, as internal processes with our pure and conscious focused attention. This is achieved as all the elements that exist outside also exist inside of us, when we cease to have any further outer desires, we simply close our *eyes, focus our attention and that becomes a reality in our experience. Once we are able to bring every process inside of us by attaining mastery of ourselves, that is considered true Pratyahara.*

Pratyahara practices lead us to a profound state of relaxation, expanded self-awareness, and inner stability. They help us master both the body and the mind. Just know this, the determination of your mind is enough, if you sit with the pure intention to go beyond our limitations to the truth of your soul, we will be guided there without a fail. Just let go, and trust that your inner being has got you. Allow yourself to flow without resistance and taste the bliss.

6 DHARANA (CONCEPTUALIZATION OR CONCENTRATION)

The name Dharana stems from a word in Sanskrit called dhri, which means to carry or to maintain.

Dharana is a noun that came about from the sanskrit word concentration of your mind by the act of holding, supporting, maintaining, retaining. Veering the space of the universe back into the space of our heart and mind is Dharana.

There are 5 types of Dharana:

First step is concentrating on a solid object which is called Vitarka, second type is Vichara or concentration on something subtle such as our senses or the mind itself, third is Ananda which means concentrating on the state of joy, forth is Asmita which means individuality and fifth would be Nirguna or concentration on nothing.

Vitarka relates to objects of concentration being in solid form associated with the activities of mind, very practically put it is visualization of any form. It can also be focusing on an idol made from a meditation mantra where in the mantra the description of the qualities would enable us to have a clear picture of the image we are looking to keep steady in our mind such as in the case of the shiva mantra.

The second one, Vichara, focuses on energy, the senses, the mind and matter. This is called Vichara, this involves concentrating on a sound, a smell, a thought, or on the subtleness of energy such as an electron.

The third, Ananda, is achieved just by the act of being happy, like concentrating on pure joy.

The fourth, Asmita, is concentrating on the individuality of the self, by being the observer of the self, mentally detaching from the body and seeing oneself as the observer.

Nirguna is the practice of concentration without an object of attention, without a thought. The mind simply stands still.

In order to enter into the Dharana state we must either focus our mind into a state of zero-ness, nothing and everything existing simultaneously, as all is source, or we can choose to focus on any form of source such as: earth, air, water, fire and space. You can focus on 1, 2 or all 5. This could be any form from nature, perhaps a tree or maybe an image of your choice such as Buddha, Krishna or Jesus. In other words, it's the initial step for deeply focused meditation, in which the object being focused upon is held in the mind without consciousness veering here and there from it. The key is focus, keeping the mind steady.

We must try to focus on the 5 elements of the universe and how they correlate to the human experience. The earth, water, fire, air and space have a close and direct relationship to us. This awareness can assist us on our journey to liberation when we can feel this bond and connection.

When deciding on what element you wish to focus upon, you can consider the following aspects to help you in the process. Each body part correlates to each universal element depending on their location. For example the corresponding body parts to the element of Earth extend from the the feet up to the knees, then from knees to the anus and genitals it's the area that correlates to the element of Water, from anus up to heart is the area related to the element of Fire, from the heart to the eyes it's the area in direct connection to the element of Air, and anything above that region corresponds to the element of Space.

The following mantras assist us in enhancing our connection and our practice: LANG for Earth, VANG for Water, RANG for Fire, YANG for Air, and HANG for Space. By simply chanting these syllables you will enhance your meditation.

When you concentrate on the earth with the sound LANG, this practice is linked to your root Chakra or Mooladhara Chakra and the god related is Lord Ganesh. You can choose to focus on this energy center or on the image of the god associated with it. It is all vibration and has the same beneficial effects.

Source exists in many forms, as the creator, the observer and the destroyer.

The creator and the creation reside within the Sacral Chakra or Swdisthana Chakra related to Water so we must focus on the sound VANG to connect with this element. It is related to the Sacral chakra and to the God Brahma, therefore you can sustain the image of running water, a waterfall perhaps or the qualities and image of this deity as both will be related to this energy center and with the use of the mantra you will easily make the connection.

The observer form of source lives within the element of Fire so focusing on the sound RANG will allow resonance with this element. It is linked to the Manipura Chakra or Solar Plexus and the God related to it is Vishnu.

The importance of life source lives within the air we breathe so focusing on music and singing, praising with the vibration YANG will connect us with our breath. VAYU which is Air is connected to the Anahata Chakra and the god related to it is Rudra which is the destroyer preparing yourself for a new creation.

Life lives within the Vissuddha or Throat Chakra and chanting HANG will make us connect with the element of Space. The god related to it is Jeeva.

The Ajna Chakra which is the third eye, will be enhanced by chanting OHM, as OHM is the sound of creation. Anyone can pronounce this sound even those who can't speak can utter this universal vibration. It is the combination of AAAHHH, UHHHH and MMMMM, this will enhance your consciousness level.

The Sahastara Chakra or Crown Chakra as we know is formless, NO form of source lives within this space so concentrating on nothingness or the stars in space for example will enhance this element in us. From consciousness you rise to nothingness.

A person who is capable of concentrating for an extended length of time of about 2 hours by inhaling and exhaling consciously, by consciously taking the air to your Root Chakra and focusing continuously on the element of earth, you will no doubt become victorious. As the element of earth is Love.

Similarly if you can concentrate on the mantra of water VANG and see yourself as the observer for a period of time of about 2 hours, you will successfully rid yourself of all ailments as water is responsible for all diseases. This is better understood when we have acknowledgement that anytime earth and water come into contact fermentation takes place therefore is breeding ground for dis-ease takes place. The idea is to inhale focusing on the element of Water, the Sacral Chakra or Brahma, hold for a minute making a sound VAN, and then exhale. Focus and intention is key, if you are capable of focusing in this manner for 2 hours you will be dis-ease free.

Third step involves the same procedure by concentrating on Fire, chanting the mantra RANG and keeping your focus on your Solar Plexus for a period of time. This practice will make you victorious over the element of fire. All those looking to lower your blood pressure, cure pneumonia, COVID-19 and other types of lack of heat should focus on this step.

For the Air mantra we must focus on the importance of source and chant YANG, then the person becomes victorious over air, at that point the person will be able to live without food and water.

If you can concentrate on space with the space mantra HANG and focus on nothing, at that point you will have become one with life, nothing will matter to you, good and bad will cease to exist for you, all opposition dies off and then your birth and death cycle are concluded forever.

7 DHYANA (MEDITATION)

Meditation is not an act, it's a state of being or quality we must embody. It is a continuous flow of the same energy, we achieve it by maintaining an image of an object of meditation without being distracted by any other thought. It is training the mind to remain concentrated and fixed on a certain internal or external quality. When you concentrate on nothingness or "nothing" "something" cannot enter the mind.

During true meditation the meditator is not conscious of the act of meditation. He or she only exists as consciousness of being, he or she is only aware of the consciousness of being. It is a process free from all distractions and awakens self awareness or higher self called Atman. That is a non afflicted, conflict-less and blissful state of freedom.

There are 2 types of Dhyana practices:

Nothing is translated as Nirgun dhyana in sanskrit. In which the meditator meditates on "nothing" or source, on pure consciousness like space.

That which is nowhere and everywhere, which is pure and beyond opposition, in the absence of words, beyond touch, beyond sight and smell and is continuous. It contains all opposites and simultaneously contains nothing.

It's nothing yet it's present everywhere as a base for everyone and all energy, the entire universe, beyond life and death. It is invisible but present in the meditator, present in earth, water, fire, and air.

It's spread everywhere it sees everyone yet no one can see it. It touches everyone but no one can touch it, it faces all directions and yet I am it.

Basically you are meditating on yourself because that is what you truly are.

Some will meditate on their Ishta (cherished divinity) or prefered god. The way in which the meditator wants to experience source or the way he wants to experience nothing or void. And then sometimes conceptualize nothing as something which can be like light present everywhere and can go everywhere in the shape of space or sky, very pure, immortal, blissful, fair, in the form of white bright light as their Ishta.

Meditating on "something" is Sagun dhyana in sanskrit. Here the object becomes the qualities and for this type of meditation you have to conceptualize your Ishta, deity or god in the form in which you wish to experience it.

There are several types and when performed take us towards Source but also provide us with some physical benefits. These health benefits are that the meditator moves forward towards attaining liberation. When we meditate on our third eye chakra the meditator attains a meditative state and rids himself of birth and death cycles. Among the Sagun dhyana practices, there is a variety you can focus on: kindness meditation, progressive meditation, mindfulness meditation, prana meditation, kundalini meditation and transcendental meditation.

Kindness meditation consists of the attitude of love towards everybody and everything even towards your enemies and sources of your stress. With every inhale we take in love and kindness and then send it to specific people and circumstances with every exhalation. It promotes feelings of love and compassion both for others and ourselves.

It enhances positive emotions and reduces anxiety and depression, it can help those who are affected by anger, frustration, resentment and interpersonal conflict.

Progressive meditation encourages us to scan a specific part of our body or areas of tension and thereby notice and allow the tension to leave the body. We must start from our feet towards our crown chakra, tensing and releasing each area of our body. If you have more than one area of tension, it will provide you with a feeling of calmness.

Mindfulness meditation is being aware and present here in the now, and not dwelling on the past or future, which is just a mis-use of the asset of your mind. It can be practiced anywhere at any time. It reduces any negative emotion, improves the focus of the mind and memory, it also enhances the feeling of satisfaction in all our relationships.

Prana meditation is a meditation practice where our awareness is solely on our breath. We breathe slowly and deeply focusing on our breath. It improves concentration, emotional flexibility, and reduces all anxiety present in the body.

Kundalini Meditation is that which blends meditation with a mantra. It provides us with physical strength, mental health and reduces depression, pain and anxiety.

Transcendental meditation is that in which the meditator remains seated in lotus, breathes slowly or does not breathe at all (hipoxia practice), it enhances and raises our current state of being.

We can turn every moment of our life into a meditative practice. We can choose to transform our present reality in any way we want. By giving it 100% focus without losing ourselves in the outer world, while releasing worries, stress and anxieties we can derive great value from the practice. The act of meditation is simply to be in the present moment within ourselves, uninvolved in the experience of our senses.

In its true form it is a state in which one cannot be disturbed by external forces as you are totally and completely within the calmness and deepness of your inner ocean and the ripples and waves of the surface cannot touch you.

8 SAMADHI (MEDITATIVE STATE)

It is the highest state of mental concentration that we can achieve during meditation, this state unites us with the highest reality and therefore it can be defined as oneness with the object of meditation. It is a state where there is no distinction between the act of meditating and the object of meditation. Samadhi is also of 2 types: the first which is supported by an object of attention called Samprajnata samadhi or Savikalpa Samadhi, and the other which is when you focus on "nothing" and you are able to connect with the life force within that is void of name or image, that part of us which is simply on and present every beating second. It is a nameless state of being where you realize there is no more learning needed, no more practices, all that IS resides within and it is active and vibrating at full capacity. This is the point where there are no words and no description can be uttered. This state is called Nirvikalpa Samadhi Nirbija.

It is oneness and unification with the object of meditation. All your needs get reduced to the point where you realize nothing in the outer world is of any importance, you go completely within and you obtain the wisdom in which you ultimately understand: All is source

Samadhi is one of the tools that takes us to enlightenment. Let's say probably the ultimate tool we master when on the path towards obtaining enlightenment and liberation.

Enlightenment means you have understood, you have obtained the wisdom to know Source, you have gained complete understanding of who you are from your beginning to your ultimate, complete knowing that what you are is nothing but consciousness. We are all a piece of this vast universe, and at the same time the whole universe resides within us, all duality ends, there is no more I like this, I don't like that. Duality ends in Samadhi.

What does this mean? The mantra that you are uttering weather guru mantra or simply ohm is one with source, you are one with source and there is complete awareness of this connection 100% of the time. Oneness means that the object of meditation, your mantra and you have become one.

When our existence is in a meditative state we become the object of meditation. We don't need to sit in lotus with your eyes closed, we can be fully functioning in the world and with your eyes open and be in a permanent meditative state of being. That is the ultimate state and it is accessible for every human being, he who observes the 8 limbs of yoga naturally obtains this. That is to become one with that which is already present in us, it can only be experienced and not described or explained therefore we invite you to experience the bliss of who you really are.

We learn the art of unification with our object of meditation through Samadhi.
This art of unification you have now mastered, you can use in your life to understand unification with Source, where the knowing that all energies reside within. That level of awareness is known as enlightenment. And that it is when the real spirituality starts, after the enlightenment state has begun.

From this point on you have understood that you are consciousness and that which is you is present in every one of us and everything, this energy comes from nothing and therefore in your oneness with nothingness, you become nothing. And that is when Liberation is possible for you.

When walking the spiritual path you need 100% commitment to transform your life. In my personal journey 2 things made it possible for me to reach liberation: making the decision at the right time and consistent practice which makes anything we do, perfect. When I tried doing yoga for the first time it was so difficult for me to sit in lotus and I wanted to obtain lotus pose as my chosen asana. I was determined and I was committed to practice daily. The first day I sat a total of 35 seconds, then slowly it started increasing. It took lots of effort, work, and will power but within 6 months I was able to completely sit for the total 32 minutes. Later other yoga asanas helped me achieve flexibility in my body by integrating my pranayama into it. I would always feel fresh and happy, determined to put in the work in my chanting and other spiritual practices without feeling laziness.

I have to add I also had 100% commitment towards my guru, this commitment to move forward kept me going. Reading books was not that helpful to be honestly, as you have now understood, it is not an intellectual process. The cleansing process was disgusting to me, but it was a necessary step in the process that would ultimately take me where I wanted to go. Which was my blending with the nothingness that is everything.

The main difference between meditation and meditative state is that meditation is done in cycles of time whereas meditative state is a permanent state of being. Time only exists when there is a distance to be traveled from point A to point B.

Here you finally realize there is no goal to attain nor any place you need to arrive at. You are already there, you have arrived.

You finally REALIZE, you never left.

A DAY IN THE LIFE OF YOGI

First Week

Wake up in Brahma Muhurta (starts around 3:30 am until sunrise)

Pray to Earth for supporting my life, be thankful to source

Morning routine

Meditation (until 5:30 am)

Asanas

Wait 1 hour before having breakfast to let energies settle

Breakfast (keep in mind to eat 50% at capacity of your stomach)

Enjoy Life (work, etc) during this time remember yamas and follow thoroughly

Lunch (keep in mind to eat 50% at capacity of your stomach)

Enjoy Life

Be Nice to your family members, hold their hands and walk a little

Eat an early dinner (2 hours before sleeping)

Pranayama (1 round) or chanting (30 min to 2 hours)

Be thankful

Go to savasana (dead body posture) between 9:30 pm and 10 pm. Do not watch anything on your TV or your phone before going to sleep.

CONCLUSION

We made it, we have studied all 8 limbs of yoga with the addition of mudras and chakras to better expand our understanding and experience. It should be clear by now that the process must be done systematically and in chronological order as we have mentioned throughout.

Yoga in the way we have discussed and learned is a way of attaining our higher self and reveals the cure for nearly every problem. It's the process by which we can transcend our limited thinking and embrace a more expansive state of being. We un-identify with our body and mind as we realize we are the intelligence that provides our body and mind with life, yet we are not them. We become aware that we are the source enabling the body with movement, and animating what would otherwise be an inanimate object, and that is a great distinction.

However this is not a one day affair, nor a magic pill. This advanced system is a way of life, it shall be performed regularly and preferably under the guidance of a spiritual teacher. The state of yoga (**unification with Source**), can only be achieved when we establish ourselves in this wisdom. "First establish yourself in yoga then act in the world", I am paraphrasing a wise Yogi.

We have covered lifestyle and have gained understanding, as our emphasis has been to bring this ancient wisdom as it was originally intended to be taught and followed, how it initially existed in the universe. We must know that what we find in the world as "yoga" nowadays has been diluted through the years to simply the exercise component, having been continuously modified by many yoga teachers. Now we present the *broader spectrum of all that it entails and what it can do for our life, when incorporated in all its splendor.*

Our goal was to bring unfiltered information, useful and easy to practice. You do not need belief in its efficacy as this is not a religion, nor a philosophy. It works simply because it is a practical system or technology available at our disposal for us to serve ourselves.

It is important to keep in mind that ultimately our goal is total detachment from all aspects of us that are not intrinsically us, we are not our body, we are not our mind, we are not the material things we possess or achievements in our life. All these things we have simply accumulated through time, nothing more, nothing less. We are the existence that supports all material life around us, yet now you have the awareness to create that space between what we truly are and what we are not, we can tap into a dimension otherwise inaccessible.

To realize that all these things in my life are mine but they are not who I AM. Letting go of anything we tend to cling onto, mostly ideas and people with whom we are heavily intertwined with, that is the objective. If we think about it, to give up petty little things really carries no meaning, but renouncing everything, that is something!

We must un-identify ourselves with our body mainly our earth and water aspect and perceive ourselves instead as an ethereal self, that is our aim. As we now know we are made up of 5 elements: Earth is the first element (food that we consume from earth that gets converted into our body). Now 10 times more important than Earth is Water (blood and all fluids in our body), 100 times more important than Water is Air (our breath), 1000 times more important than water is Fire (as it maintains our body temperature) but most important is space, the ethereal part of us, without it, life would cease to exist.

Logical minds will argue about the beginning of time as they believe life started with the big bang and that nothing existed prior to it. But there is a flaw in this premise, even if you adhere to this theory, clearly there was a force responsible for the big bang, the only truth is that all life is continuous, the universe is Sanatana (continuous) and therefore there is no beginning and no end.

All wisdom is available when we tap into a certain level of frequency in the universe which exists in the form of entropy. And...What is entropy? It is the energy that doesn't get converted into work, it stays unfeathered and permanently remains in the universe for the rest of time in its original vibrational form. The scriptures call this everlasting energy vedas, it's the vibrating frequency in the universe where all truth resides. When we are capable of entering into the meditative state we vibrate at the same frequency of this energy and as we reach the awakening stage we get connected to this wisdom. Every answer can be found in the universe if we vibrate at this level, and we are able to download the cosmos into ourselves as we are one and the same.

*Nothing is known to us about the future and it's not even important. Important is how we **react in any given situation** in the present moment, not worrying about the past or future. That is what lies in our hands. Our higher self will take care of us and provide us with all the health, abundance and wealth we desire, if we live in alignment with it. Feeling good should be our single priority, it will boost our own health and will spread hope, love and light.*

The desire and need to control the future is ego-based. We cut or pinch ourselves off from source by a lack of faith and divine communion, as we are not resonating with our highest vibration. Be afraid of nothing. Place source's constant presence in our consciousness – knowing that we are always taken care of. We allow blessings to reach us faster when we are in a relaxed and aligned state of mind, that does not long to control anything.

So lets be very pragmatic about this book and the use of this wisdom in our daily lives, let's say we have a goal. At this initial phase the chances of us achieving that goal are close to zero as there has been no conscious step towards achieving this goal, we have just come to awareness of *what we want. In that instant we must simply and unequivocally make the single conscious decision, that is "No Matter What, I will succeed", without a doubt, full knowing and complete conviction. Trusting that the universe has heard us and has our back. Even if at this point it's still unbeknownst to us how the invisible forces of the cosmos will conspire to help us, IT WILL HAPPEN. There is nothing off limits, nothing so great that cannot come into our experience. We are one with creation, and we must have absolute and resolute knowing of this. This brings undoubted wisdom. Just by this conscious act you have achieved 50% of the goal, now the remaining 50% is the work we put into the **8 limbs of yoga** which makes any objective and goal attainable and achievable! Now, THAT IS POWERFUL, that is being one and the same with Source.*

BE WELL, BE HAPPY, BE CONNECTED.

Printed in the United States
by Baker & Taylor Publisher Services